SHARE THE FIRE

Dr. Guy Chevreau served the Baptist Church from 1979 to 1994. With a B.A. in philosophy, and a Masters of Divinity from Acadia Divinity College, he received his Th.D. from Wycliffe College, Toronto School of Theology, having studied in the area of historical theology. In September of 1994, he became part of the renewal team based at the Toronto Airport Christian Fellowship. Part of the time, he teaches at the morning pastors' and leaders' sessions held throughout the week; about half of most months, he serves international conferences as part of TACF's renewal team.

Guy is the author of *Catch the Fire*, which sets what has come to be known as the "Toronto Blessing" in some biblical and historical context, and complements these studies with present-day testimonies of the impartation of God's grace and love that hundreds of thousands have received through this remarkable outpouring of the Spirit. Since its release in October '94, *Catch the Fire* has been translated into nine foreign languages.

Pray With Fire serves as a sequel; its subtitle is "Interceding in the Spirit." While there are several books that encourage us to pray *for* revival, no other addresses what it means to pray *in the midst* of an outpouring of God's Spirit. And rather than spelling out another methodology for prayer, this book is a call to an ever-deepening relationship with the Lord Who wants to speak to us more than we want to speak with Him. In his review, Dr. John White said, "This book spells the difference between praying with fire and playing with it."

Guy is married to Janis; they have two children, Graham and Caitlin. When it's windy enough, Guy is likely to be found out in Lake Ontario, windsurfing.

"I count myself one of the number of those who
write as they learn
and learn as they write."

Augustine, *Letters.*[1]

[1] Nicene and Post Nicene Fathers, vol.I, Hendrickson Pub. 1994, p.490.

Guy Chevreau

SHARE THE FIRE
The Toronto Blessing
And Grace Based Evangelism

Preface by John Arnott, Senior Pastor of the Toronto
Airport Christian Fellowship

Unless otherwise indicated, all Scripture citations are from the Revised English Bible.

Canadian Cataloguing in Publication Data

Chevreau, Guy
   Share the fire : the Toronto Blessing and grace based evangelism

Includes bibliographical references.
ISBN 0-9681642-0-X

1. Evangelistic work. 2. Grace (Theology). 3. Religious awakening - Christianity. 4. Toronto Airport Christian Fellowship. I. Title.

BV3777.C3C453 1996   269'.2'09713541   C96-932462-6

Printed in Canada

CONTENTS

PREFACE

Three years after the initial outbreak of Revival in our Toronto Church, many of us have had opportunity to have significant involvement in nurturing, spreading and sharing the fire of God, not only in our own back yard, but in numerous nations and denominations around the world. We have seen a tiny flame grow into a vast and glorious "forest fire" for the Kingdom of God. As God has poured out His Spirit, so many people have received what we call "the Father's Blessing."

Dr. Guy Chevreau is one who has traveled the globe during this time, sharing his delightful and powerful insights with the Body of Christ, with those who are hungry and eager not only to learn more, but also to surrender their lives in this great move of the Holy Spirit. His first book, *Catch the Fire* has served so well to introduce many leaders and laymen alike to the intensity of the Holy Spirit's ministry and the physical manifestations that so often accompany His presence. Guy has so served us in demonstrating that the manifestations we see today are so very similar to those that characterized historical revivals of previous centuries; with his grounding in the Scriptures, he has always pointed beyond the manifestations, and helped us to focus on the abundance of good fruit.

In his second book, *Pray With Fire*, Guy helped resource us further, as we attend to what the Spirit continuously calls forth from us. It was sobering to learn that it has always been revivals' best friends that have killed things! To surrender our agendas, and discern what is on God's has been one of our foremost concerns these last three years.

Guy's study of revelatory ministry has also served us well, for the release of prophetic giftings is one of the key dynamics to all that the Lord purposes in this outpouring.

As we have talked, Guy and I agree that the greatest and most needed revelation that must come to the Church is that of the Father's great love for us, individually as well as corporately. Eternal life, and indeed everything we receive from the Father is His gift of grace. It is expressed through Christ's saving and healing love, which cannot be earned, deserved, or bought. It is nothing of works, lest any should boast. (Ephesians 2.8-9) Rather, it is a love that sets the captives free. It is the very nature and heart of the Father to freely give of Himself and His blessings to those of us who are least deserving.

I remember the time that I did not realize the full significance of the word "grace." To me it sounded like a term other religions would use; or something that theologians would talk about. It was a "Christianese" word that was often heard yet seldom understood. It was revelation to me when I learned that the word simply means "gift," from *charis* in ancient Greek.

This free gift of grace is the foundation of Dr. Chevreau's new book *Share the Fire*. Again Guy has served us as he addresses one of the questions we are most frequently asked: "Where is all of this going?" We believe that our Father purposes the greatest ingathering of souls that the world has ever seen. The Lord of the Harvest has waited patiently for His harvest to come in, and there will be a grace based evangelism that goes into the highways and byways and compels the lost to come in. It truly is "Amazing Grace."

This book will help equip you and encourage you to believe that our God, Who is mighty to save, wants now to reap the earth (Rev. 14:16). With great anticipation for an imminent and unprecedented harvest, I heartily recommend this work to you.

John Arnott
Pastor
Toronto Airport Christian Fellowship

ACKNOWLEDGEMENTS

It has been two years and one month since I sent *Catch the Fire* off to HarperCollins. In Sydney, Australia, I received a prophetic word of encouragement that the Lord purposed three books in two years – with the completion of *Share the Fire*, that word has come to pass. My Heavenly Father has been so very faithful, and so incredibly gracious to me.

What a tremendous privilege to be part of this move of God's Spirit! It has literally swept the earth these last thirty-four months, and as the Lord has called me round to fifteen different countries, and over fifty different cities, I am so grateful to my hosts – they have been some of the most godly, humble, obedient, generous, and Christ-like men and women I have ever had the pleasure of meeting. So many have become such very good friends. Thank you for your love and acceptance.

To those who are freely giving away what they have freely received, those who are sharing good news with the poor, and serving the outcasts, and befriending the stranger, and caring for the fatherless, I bless you in the name of Jesus. It has been an honour to walk with you, even for the briefest of moments. Thank you to all those who released their testimonies for publication.

The Toronto Airport Christian Fellowship is our home church. Our debt of gratitude there is immense. To the staff, both pastoral and support, as well as to the church Body – the words "thank you" are impoverished.

On the home front, it feels as though we've shifted from one unexpectedly extended sprint, and begun to pace things for a longer run. So much has changed for us as a family. Janis, Graham and Caitlin, I cannot say it often enough: you are cherished and precious gifts. I love you so much.

Final thanks go to Dr. Barry Morrison – your critical comments on the drafts helped sharpen the focus. To Alan Wiseman – again, bless you for your faithful intercessions and prophetic encouragement.

Oakville, Ontario
October, 1996

J.J.

CHAPTER ONE

SUCH SHOUTING AND JUMPING, IT SETS ME TO DOUBTING:

A Prologue

No place is left for any human pride in the presence of God. By God's act you are in Christ Jesus; God has made Him our wisdom, our holiness, our liberation. Therefore, in the words of Scripture, 'If anyone should boast, let him boast in the Lord.' 1 Corinthians 1.29-31

* * *

On July 10th, 1996, a twenty-five-year-old named Bobby[1] walked into the foyer of the Toronto Airport Christian Fellowship. Bobby had lived on the streets since he was twelve, and had been using and dealing drugs for the last fourteen years. He met his Hell's Angel father for the first time when he was eighteen. His life was, as he described it, "getting high, robbing people, and hurting people." For the last five years, Bobby had been in jail for Christmas. He is functionally illiterate.

---

[1] Because of his recent conversion, pastoral staff felt it wisest to use a pseudonym.

1

This particular afternoon, he was high on crack cocaine and marijuana, and had a loaded gun in his pocket. Needing money for drugs, he had come to rob the place. Bobby had misunderstood the name of the church, and because of some misinformation, he thought that it was an Italian card and casino club – he figured he'd soon have in his pocket the poker money he expected to steal.

Sandy, the foyer receptionist, was the first one to speak to him. As she looked at him as he walked in, she had a feeling that he was so very lost, and that he desperately needed to know the Father's love. Bobby said that just standing in the foyer, he was overwhelmed with what he now knows to be the presence of God; what he knew initially was that his drug buzz evaporated. As Sandy and Bobby talked, she invited him to the evening meeting. He said, "You wouldn't want my kind here." She asked why. He answered, "I'm a criminal." Sandy assured him that he was more than welcome. He responded that there wasn't any hope for him, and that his family had given up on him. Again, Sandy invited him to the meeting, feeling an urgency to say something more. She looked into his eyes, and said, "God really loves you." Bobby was stunned, and became choked up with tears; he panicked, and headed back out the door.

Outside, he sat down on the curb, his head in his hands. Some time later, a man came and sat beside him. They talked; Bobby had tears in his eyes; the man also

2

suggested that he come to the meeting later that night. Bobby got some sleep behind one of the local warehouses, and after he had smoked a couple of joints to bolster his courage, he made his way into the meeting. That night, when the salvation call was issued, he gave his life to Jesus. Hours later, as he had done so many other nights, he slept on a picnic bench.

Over the course of the next month, Bobby was befriended by and incorporated into the young adults group at the church, and began to be discipled. Several of them stood with him through his bail hearing; others helped him find work, and still others are helping him manage his money. He stayed with one of the pastors for three weeks until other accommodation could be arranged, and new friends have come alongside as he re-orients his drug-free living.

On August 17th, Bobby publicly proclaimed his faith in Jesus Christ as his Saviour and Lord in the waters of baptism. When asked what are some of the changes he has noticed since his conversion, Bobby quickly answered: "I'm a hundred percent different. Instead of take, I give. I believe in the Lord; He's my God, He's number one in my life, and He's the One looking after me. The drugs are gone, the alcohol is gone, the violence is gone.... All that stuff is gone; I'm a new person; it's great."

As of October 1996, Bobby was off to Teen Challenge, a Christian drug rehabilitation program, for a year of discipleship. Upon graduation, he hopes to go back to the streets to share the love of God with the homeless.

* * *

The vast majority of those visiting the Toronto Airport Christian Fellowship have come with markedly different motives than Bobby's. But many have been met no less dramatically. *The Toronto Star's* Faith and Ethics newspaper reporter began her story on the second "Catch the Fire" conference, held in October 1995:

"The mighty winds of hurricane Opal that swept through Toronto last week were mere tropical gusts compared with the power of God thousands believe struck them senseless at a conference of the controversial Airport Vineyard Church."

She continued:

At least with Opal, they could stay on their feet. Not so with many of the 5,300 souls meeting at the Regal Constellation Hotel. The ballroom carpets were littered with fallen bodies, bodies of seemingly straight-laced men and women, who felt themselves moved by the phenomenon they say is the Holy Spirit. So moved, they howled with joy or the release of some long buried pain. They collapsed, some rigid as corpses, some convulsed in hysterical

4

laughter. From room to room come barnyard cries, calls heard only in the wild, grunts so deep women recalled the sounds of childbirth, while some men and women adopted the very position of childbirth.[2]

Four months later, the Toronto Airport Christian Fellowship was again in the headlines: *The post-Toronto phenomenon – when have we laughed enough and can go back to work?*

Most of the churches worldwide which have been affected by the Toronto-phenomenon are going through a phase of re-orientation. The attitude of most pastors we meet is "We tried it, it didn't hurt, but it didn't help much either." Beside the many positive reports in the areas of counseling, self-discovery and honesty, and the extremely few reports in the areas of evangelization and mission, there is now a fear growing in many churches that "the Toronto phenomenon" could become institutionalized.

Many blessings have died as people tried to control it, organize it or to manipulate it to fit their personal beliefs. The Bible has no problems with people falling over, but it values more what they do when they stand up again.

[2] Leslie Scrivener, *The Toronto Star*, October 8, 1995, p.A2.

> Whether we rest in the spirit [sic] or our flesh, there are still three billion completely unreached people in the world, of which the majority is under 15, people under the poverty line and in slums waiting to hear the gospel.
>
> Let's go together – as blessed as possible – to bring them this blessing.[3]

The "Toronto Blessing" has received a great deal of media attention from both secular and religious sources. The two clips above are suggestive of the diverse ways in which many are reacting. Those outside the Church are characteristically intrigued with such dynamic happenings taking place in the lives of people whom the press have tended to marginalize, if not ignore. Many inside the Church have misunderstood and even misrepresented this outpouring of God's Spirit, as in the *Island Herald* article, referring to the Blessing as "it."

But the powerful, loving presence of God is not an "it." John Arnott, the senior pastor of the Toronto Airport Christian Fellowship, continually pushes this to the forefront, even titling his book, *The Father's Blessing*. The "Heart" of what hundreds of thousands have discovered is that the Master and Creator of the Universe has chosen to reveal Himself as tender, gracious and merciful; He has come, at His own initiative, seeking the likes of us; He continuously lays

---

[3] *The Island Herald*, Victoria BC, February, 1996.

blessing over the cursedness of our lives; and He invites us into an ever-deepening relationship with Himself. This revelation is the very Gospel of Jesus Christ. In any given moment, the personal and corporate life transformations that result are at the core of Christian faith, regardless of the physical posture one assumes. The falling, and the other physical manifestations characterizing this move of the Spirit have been provocative, at very least.

Introduction to the Toronto Blessing

While a major conference like the one described in October is hosted about every other month, regular meetings are held six nights a week at the Toronto Airport Christian Fellowship (prior to January 20th, 1996, the name of the church was the Toronto Airport Vineyard). These meetings were initiated when a Vineyard pastor, Randy Clark of St. Louis, was invited to preach over a long weekend, the 20th January 1994.

Nightly congregations at the TACF average between seven to twelve hundred per night, and are drawn from literally every corner of the globe and virtually every denomination of the Body of Christ. Over 50,000 pastors have come from all over continental North America, Britain, Germany, Iceland, Scandinavia, the Netherlands, Switzerland, Austria, France, Spain, Italy, South Africa, Nigeria, Kenya, East Africa, Swaziland, Korea, Indonesia, Mongolia, Japan, New Zealand and Australia, Chile, Peru, Argentina, Guatemala,

Nicaragua.... As those on pilgrimage, they have come to receive what the British secular press nicknamed "the Toronto Blessing."

Those who have come spiritually hungry have experienced a depth of spiritual refreshment, awakening, and release such that they are quick to testify that they have experienced a much needed measure of God's grace, and have seen the power of His love, demonstrated and appropriated in personal ways. Thousands of defeated, discouraged and exhausted Christians have testified that through the Blessing, they've never known so much of God's love for them, nor known so much love for Him. Many have experienced a renewing of commitment and call, an enlarging and clarification of spiritual vision, and a rekindled passion for Jesus and the work of the Kingdom. Thousands of desperate and burned-out pastors and their spouses have been refreshed, re-commissioned, and released in new freedom, authority and power to declare the good news of Jesus Christ.

But it has not just been believers who have formed the nightly congregations. While problematic to track, the New Life ministry teams have made contact with at least 8,000 prodigals who have come forward for prayer as they re-commit their lives; over 6,000 have made first-time professions of faith. Bobby was one of these.

These are the more consequential dynamics at work in "the Toronto Blessing." What has generated so much of the attention are the physical manifestations that have often accompanied this gracious outpouring of God's Spirit – hysterical laughter, shouting, shaking, and the like. These phenomena have caused some to take such exception to the Toronto "Blessing" that they call this movement the "Toronto Blasphemy." Such critics are adamant that God does not "do" these sorts of things to His people. However, a close reading of primary records of past, *bona-fide* revivals indicates many striking similarities to much of the phenomena that have come to characterize what the guarded have alternatively called the "Toronto Mixed Blessing."

Wisdom does not judge what it does not understand

As I have continued to research past moves of God, my pre-renewal characterization of historic revivals has been challenged. The typical picture of the Welsh revival, for example, is that of the coal miners coming straight from the pit to chapel, their blackened faces soon washed with free-flowing tears of repentance. However, a closer, and more comprehensive study of the historical record seems to indicate strong precedent for much of what is being experienced by so many as they find themselves "Toronto Blessed." Grawys Jones, a local pastor of Aberdare, Wales, spoke of his experience in the early days of the 1904-5 revival:

> Some most strange joy took possession of the whole congregation. The only way I can describe it is this – as if a great shower were

9

coming down the valley here – I have seen it often – and you can hear the noise of it in the wind, and then by and by a few big drops come, the forerunner of the great shower. Exactly like that it came. I knew that something great was approaching.

Jones described how as the man who was leading in prayer closed, another started singing, and as the congregation lifted their praise for a quarter of an hour,

some were shouting for joy, and others praying. We three ministers in the pulpit were crying for joy, the tears running down our faces. We were lost to everything, and forgot all about this world, I think. The joy of it, the immense, untold joy of it was something that I never, never dreamed possible....

That particular meeting went late into the night.

About 4 o'clock (in the morning) I went home, and I could hear companies in the early morning singing away with all their might. I went to bed but could hardly sleep, and when I did I was laughing for joy in my sleep, and I got up in the morning full of joy.[4]

[4] Brynmor Jones, *Voices from the Welsh Revival 1904-1905*. Evangelical Press of Wales, p.174.

Such an account is not an isolated mutation of true revival. Written fifty-six years earlier (1848), the following is a dialogue song between a "Shouting" Methodist and a "Formalist," most likely either a Presbyterian or a Congregationalist. It is a graphic description of the meetings conducted, and reflects a most remarkable similarity to the experience of "Toronto's" friends and sceptics, both the questions raised and the answers given.

The Methodist begins with warm greeting:
"Good morning, brother pilgrim! What, trav'ling to Zion?
What doubts and what dangers have you met today?
Have you gain'd a blessing, then pray without ceasing,
Press forward, my brother and make no delay;
Have you a desire that burns like a fire,
And long for the hour when Christ shall appear?"

The Formalist responds by describing his experience at the Methodist's meetings:
"I came out this morning, and now I'm returning,
Perhaps little better than when I first came,
Such groaning and shouting, it sets me to doubting,
I fear such religion is only a dream.
The preachers are stamping, the people are jumping,
And screaming so loud that I nothing could hear,
Either the praying or preaching – such horrible shrieking!
I was truly offended at all that was there."

The Methodist asks after the Formalist's involvement:
"Perhaps, my dear brother, while they prayed together
You sat and considered, but prayed not at all:
Would you find a blessing, then pray without ceasing,
Obey the advice that was given by Paul.
For if you should reason at any such season,
No wonder if Satan should tell in your ear,
That preachers and people are only a rabble,
And this is no place for reflection and prayer."

The Formalist recoils:
"No place for reflection – I'm filled with distraction,
I wonder that people could bear for to stay,
The men they were bawling, the women were squalling,
I know not for my part how any could pray.
Such horrid confusion – if this be religion
I'm sure that it's nothing that never was seen,
For the sacred pages that speak of all ages,
Do nowhere declare that such ever has been."

The Methodist takes over with his apologetic:
"Don't be so soon shaken – if *I'm* not mistaken
Such things *were* perform'd by believers of old;
When the ark was coming, King David came running,
And dancing before it, in Scripture we're told.
When the Jewish nation had laid the foundation,
To rebuild the temple at Ezra's command,
Some wept and some praised, such noise there was raised,
'Twas heard afar off and perhaps through the land....

The Formalist counters:
"Then Scripture's contrasted, for Paul has protested
That *order* should reign in the house of the Lord,
Amid such a clatter who knows what's the matter?
Or who can attend unto what is declared?
To see them behaving like drunkards, all raving,
And lying and rolling prostrate on the ground,
I really feel awful, and sometimes felt fearful
That I'd be the next that would come tumbling down."

The Methodist gives the following counsel:
"You say you felt awful – you ought to be careful
Lest you grieve the Spirit, and so He depart,
By your own confession, you've felt some impression,
The sweet melting showers have softened your heart.
You fear persecution, and that's a delusion
Brought in by the devil to stop up your way.
Be careful, my brother, for blest are no other
Than persons that 'are not offended in Me.'"

As Peter was preaching, and bold in his teaching,
The Spirit descended and some were offended,
And said of these men, 'They're filled with new wine.'
I never yet doubted that some of them shouted,
While others lay prostrate, by power struck down;
Some weeping, some praising, while others were saying:
'They're drunkards or fools, or in falsehood abound....'"

He offers to pray for the Formalist, that his "precious

soul would be filled with the fire of God."

How does it end? The Formalist is won over, confident that at very least, God's "mercy is sure unto all that believe." His testimony?

"My heart is now glowing! I feel His love flowing! Peace, pardon, and comfort I now do receive!"[5]

Share The Fire

God has continuously renewed and revived His people, both throughout the pages of the Scriptures, and in the ongoing history of His Church. This restoring work has always had a two-fold consequence of quality and quantity. Through the "Toronto Blessing," there are thousands of believers world-wide who testify to a deeper, fuller revelation of the Father's loving heart such that a new measure of faith and faithfulness has been awakened within the Church. Perhaps as never before, many recognize the truth declared by the Welsh revivalist, Evan Roberts when he said, "God cannot do a great work *through* you without doing a great work *in* you first."[6] Having been the subjects of the Lord's gracious work, there has been a broader, out-going revelation of God's love, demonstrated by those who have been revived. Put simply, we more than recognize that God pours out His Spirit not just that we "be

---

[5] Winthrop Hudson, *Encounter*, Winter 1968, vol.29, p.74.
[6] Brynmor Pierce Jones, *An Instrument of Revival: the Complete Life of Evan Roberts, 1878-1951*. Bridge Publishing: South Plainfield, NJ, 1995, p.65.

blessed," but that we "be a blessing." Writing roughly 850 years ago, the great revival preacher Bernard of Clairvaux put things this way:

[The Spirit's] operation in us is twofold. For He not only fortifies us interiorly with virtues, unto our own salvation, but He also adorns us exteriorly with His gifts, unto the salvation of others. The former are bestowed upon us for our own sakes, the latter with a view to our neighbour's advantage. For instance, we obtain faith, hope, and charity for ourselves, ... and the word of wisdom and knowledge, the grace of healing, the gift of prophecy, and the like, ... which are communicated to be employed in promoting the spiritual interests of others.[7]

* * *

The sub-title of this book is *The Toronto Blessing and Grace Based Evangelism.* As thousands of refreshed and renewed pastors, leaders and churches around the world attend to what the Spirit of the Lord is imparting and calling forth, there is the recognition that unless "streams of living water"[8] flow out from

[7] *St. Bernard's Sermons on the Canticle of Canticles*, vol.I., "On the Two Operations of the Holy Ghost." Dublin: Browne and Nolan, 1920, pgs. 174-5.
[8] John 7.38.

within, they will soon stagnate, or even recede. This recognition, however, could call forth a striving on our part that would compromise the Lord's purposes in this fresh outpouring of His Spirit. If we were to work the metaphor Jesus used in John 7, it is not we who make the stream flow out. We are the recipients of the living water that flows through us with such a super abundance that there is a wonderful overflow.

The following chapter is a consideration of some of the dynamics at work in the development of historic revivals. When studied, a general pattern and process can be discerned: believers and churches were first awakened; in turn, unbelievers came to faith in Jesus Christ, were incorporated into His Body, and used to draw others to newness of life. As with *Catch The Fire* and *Pray With Fire,* the subsequent chapters bring biblical study, historic precedent and present testimony to bear, with the view to welding Kingdom theology, mission, and an outpouring of God's Spirit together. As essentials are clarified and restated, it is hoped that the following resources and reflections will serve to help us to steward this precious anointing. With the grace of God ever before us, we recognize again that the way on is the same as the way in. Living out this Gospel revelation, we are released and empowered to share with others the fire with which we have been baptized. As such, we will be "firepots in the woodlands, and blazing torches among the sheaves."[9]

[9] Zechariah 12.6.

CHAPTER TWO

RIPPLES ON THE POND:

The Dynamics of Revival

'O man, can these bones live?' 'Only You, Lord God, know that.' '... Prophecy to the wind, prophecy, O man, and say to it: These are the words of the Lord God: Let winds come from every quarter and breathe into these slain, that they may come to life....' Ezekiel 37.3 and 9

＊ ＊ ＊

In the pastors and leaders sessions we host at the Toronto Airport Christian Fellowship, the question is repeatedly raised: "When does all of this move from renewal to revival?" Here, a word of explanation is required. The term *renewal* was suggested in the early weeks of the meetings at the Toronto Airport Vineyard, for it was felt that it would be presumptuous to name things *revival* from the start. The dynamic consequences of the protracted meetings were for history to evaluate and name. There were others who insisted that the term revival cannot be used until mass conversions are witnessed.

Definitions are critical things. Once named, they become determinative, for they set boundaries, and distinguish one thing from another. Classically, a "revival of religion" has been defined as

> the awakening into more active and living energy those religious feelings, habits, and principles, which previously existed, but which had sunk into comparative dormancy. But that is not all its meaning. It is employed also to indicate the conversion of sinners, who were previously in a state of irreligion altogether.... Revival is to be understood as an unusual manifestation of the power of the grace of God in convincing and converting careless sinners, and in quickening and increasing the faith and piety of believers.... It is the life-giving, light-imparting, quickening, regenerating, and sanctifying energy of the Holy Spirit....[1]

More recently, Donald McGavran's interpretation of revival may surprise some readers. (McGavran is the author of the "classic" text, *Understanding Church Growth,* and is considered by many as the father of the church growth movement.) He begins by quoting Edwin Orr on "awakening":

> An Evangelical Awakening is a movement of

[1]*The Revival of Religion: Addresses by Scottish Evangelical Leaders, delivered in Glasgow, 1840.* The Banner of Truth Trust, 1840/1984, Camelot Press, Southampton, p.x.

the Holy Spirit *in the Church of Christ* bringing about a revival of New Testament Christianity. Such an awakening may change in a significant way an individual only; or it may affect a larger group of people; or it may move a congregation, or the churches of a city or district, or the whole body of believers throughout the world. Such an awakening may run its course briefly, or it may last a whole lifetime.

McGavran goes on to define revival as

God's gift. Human beings can neither command it nor make God grant it. God sovereignly gives revival when and where He wills. It "breaks out," "strikes," "quickens a church," "comes with the suddenness of a summer storm," "makes its appearance," "inaugurates a work of grace," and "blesses His people".... By the very structure of the word, revival means revivification of an existing church or existing Christians. There must be first tired believers before they can be revived. All accounts tell of cold, indifferent, or sinful congregations that, by revival, are kindled to new consecration.... If the significant meaning of the word – vitalizing an existing church – is to be preserved, it must not be used for the original turnings of non-Christians to Christ.[2]

Historically, a "quickening and increase" of faith is often seen first in the church's leadership. Revival scholar Iain Murray documents the "striking change" people saw in their preachers as they were "awakened." For example, the ministry of the Presbyterian pastor, William Graham, of Lexington Virginia, was described as both "able and orthodox." While at the revival meetings that were sweeping the Blue Ridge Mountains in August 1789, Graham "was as a man suddenly transformed." In his subsequent preaching, there was a recognized increase in authority, warmth and joy. So too, with John Blair Smith, who was described as "a popular preacher,... but for years, his preaching seemed to take no effect, there was no awakening of sinners, no arousing of cold professors (believers), nor reclaiming of backsliders. But at the commencement of the great revival of 1786/7, he underwent a remarkable change in his own feelings and in the fervency of his preaching so that he became one of the most powerful preachers I ever heard."[3] The same is said of the change that came

---

[2] Donald McGavran, *Understanding Church Growth, 3rd ed.* Grand Rapids, Mich., Eerdmans Pub. Co., 1990, pgs. 134, 135 and 139. Italics added.

[3] Iain H. Murray, *Revival and Revivalism: The Making and Marring of American Evangelicalism 1750 - 1858*. The Banner of Truth Trust, 1994, Edinburgh, *p.107*.

over the Rev. Dr. John McDonald, a Scottish revival preacher:

> There have been instances of persons becoming 'other men' who were never new creatures in Christ; but there have been also instances of renewed men becoming other men under a fresh baptism of the Spirit. This was the change which Mr McDonald underwent in Edinburgh. It was soon apparent in his preaching. Always clear and sound in his statements of objective truth, his preaching had now become instinct with life. It was now searching and fervent, as well as sound and lucid.... His statements of gospel truth were now the warm utterances of one who deeply felt its power. The Lord's people could now testify that he spoke from his own heart to theirs.

Murray concludes the chapter with this assessment:

> The Great Revival taught the Presbyterian churches that orthodoxy and correct preaching, indispensable though they are, are not enough. Authority, tenderness, compassion, pity – these must be given in larger measure from heaven, and when they are it can truly be said that theology has taken fire.... The facts are

indisputable. A considerable body of men, for a long period before the Second Great Awakening, preached the same message as they did during the revival but with vastly different consequences - the same men, the same actions, performed with the same abilities, yet the results were so amazingly different![4]

The First Link in the Chain of Grace

To use McGavran's terms, there has come through the "Toronto Blessing" a most remarkable "revivification of existing Christians and churches." While there is no possible way of knowing how many individuals have formed the evening congregations, over one million people have cumulatively attended the Toronto Airport Christian Fellowship, as of May 1996. This milestone marked the fact that thousands and thousands of pastors, leaders and believers from around the world have been refreshed, renewed and awakened. Historically, this is the precursor, the forerunner, to what most understand as "classic" revival. For instance, when the Great Awakening first began in Northampton, conversions were recorded, but the most predominant awakening was that of the church. In his *A Faithful Narrative of the Surprising Work of God in the Conversion of Many Hundred Souls in Northampton*

---

[4] *Ibid*, pgs. 109 and 127.

and the Neighbouring Towns ... Jonathan Edwards noted that in late December, 1734, "the Spirit of God began to extraordinarily set in," and five or six persons were "savingly converted, some of them wrought upon in a very remarkable manner." Referring to the restorative prophecy in Ezekiel 37.1-14, he goes on to say that such glorious work caused a stir within the church: "the noise amongst the dry bones waxed louder and louder;" by the summer of 1735, this work of God had made "a glorious alteration in the town, such that it seemed to be full of the presence of God." He states: "Those among us who had been formerly converted, were greatly enlivened, and renewed with fresh and extraordinary [experiences] of the Spirit of God; though some much more than others, according to the measure of the gift of Christ. Many who had laboured under difficulties about their own [spiritual] state, now had their doubts removed by more satisfying experience, and more clear discoveries of God's love."[5]

He says of the preaching,

> the arguments are the same that they have heard hundreds of times; but the force of the arguments, and their conviction by them, is altogether new; they come with a new and before unexperienced power. Before, they

[5] *The Collected Works of Jonathan Edwards*. Edinburgh: The Banner of Truth Trust, 1992, I.348ab.

heard it was so, and they allowed it to be so;
but now they see it to be so indeed.... Persons
after their conversions often speak of religious
things as seeming new to them; that preaching
is a new thing; that it seems to them they never
heard preaching before; that the Bible is a new
book; they find there new chapters, new
psalms, new histories, because they see them
in a new light. [6]

Along with this internal awakening within the church,
Edwards conservatively estimated that in the first six
months of the revival, 300 souls were "savingly brought
home to Christ."

Joseph Tracy carefully studied the Great Awakening
one hundred years after its occurrence. He describes the
congregations that gathered to hear Edwards preach his
extended sermon series on justification by faith:

The preacher had before him a considerable
number of men, who were in no respect
regarded or treated as regenerate persons;
who were regarded, both by the church and by
themselves, as unrenewed, impenitent men,
destitute of faith, and of every Christian grace,
and in the broad road to perdition. It was not
merely feared or believed that the

[6] *Ibid.*, I.356ab.

congregation contained many such persons.
The church records contained the names of
those who were supposed to be in the road to
heaven; and others were, by common consent,
to be regarded and addressed as persons in the
road to hell.

The theological backdrop to this situation was that a
pragmatic Arminianism had been taught for years – such
that well-intentioned, but unconverted men and women
believed that they could, without supernatural grace,
live an ethical and social life that would be pleasing to
God, and that those who were doing so, were doing
very well. Edwards made it clear that the gravity of sin,
and the peril of an uncertain profession of faith in
Christ's saving grace made such "works righteousness"
a spiritual folly. Of the results of Edwards' passionate
preaching, Tracy brings forward the following critical
assessments:

Great numbers of church members were
converted. We must remember that the
practice of admitting to the communion all
persons neither heretical nor scandalous, was
general in the Presbyterian church, and
prevailed extensively among the
Congregational churches. In consequence, a
large proportion of the communicants in both
were unconverted persons. Multitudes of these

were converted.... In some cases, the revival seems to have been almost wholly within the church, and have resulted in the conversion of nearly all the members.... These converted church members, from want of their piety, were at best dead weights to the churches. They now became active and valuable members.

There was a twofold gain In every such instance, the church felt its encumbering burden diminished, and its strength increased.[7]

History Repeats Itself

Similar dynamics are traced in a subsequent move of the Spirit. Prior to the Second Great Awakening, church life in general was described as "cold and dead." In 1760, churches of Baptist persuasion were "few in number and of negligible influence." One Virginian Christian declared, "too many Presbyterians were sound in doctrine but deficient in experience."[8] In the early years of 1800, God graciously poured out His Spirit, especially through camp meetings like the ones held in Cane Ridge, Kentucky. The situation *slowly, but dynamically*, began to change. Of the estimated 10,000 people in the meetings in August of 1801, 144 conversions were recorded – a fairly small yield.

[7] Joseph Tracy, *The Great Awakening: A History of the Revival. . .* Edinburgh: The Banner of Truth Trust, 1842/1989, pgs. 4, 391-2.
[8] Iain Murray, *Op. cit.*, pgs. 65 and 93.

However, a local Baptist church nearby had added only 6 to the church in the five years that preceded the outpouring, but two years after the summer meetings, that one fellowship added 320 new members. A sister church had been static for 19 years; in the two years following the camp meetings, they baptized 318 new believers. The nearby Elkhorn Association of Baptist Churches was made up of 27 churches, and, in 1800, had 1642 members. Two years after the outpouring, 21 new churches had begun, membership having more than tripled.

Thirty, Sixty, a Hundred Fold

These statistics are only to demonstrate the exponential, slowly starting, but dynamically gaining growth patterns in revival. This is exactly the description of the growth pattern of the Kingdom, as Jesus said it would be in teachings such as the parables of the sower, the mustard seed, and the leaven.[9] There is, as it were, botanical progression here. God releases a fresh outpouring of gifts, resources, and a dynamic empowerment for ministry, but these take some time to "take root" before they "bear fruit." In terms of evangelism, this is especially the case. One unbeliever comes to Christ and is nurtured in his or her faith. Over the next weeks and months, this zealous evangelist witnesses to unchurched family and friends. As they see

[9] Matthew 13.8, 32 and 33.

the qualitative life transformation evidenced as the new believer lives his or her life in Christ, there is a credible and dynamic witness which leads to further conversions, sometimes of whole families and friendship networks.

In 1770 there were fewer than a thousand American Methodists. By 1820, fifty years later, there were over two hundred and fifty thousand. There was both remarkable spiritual growth and a tremendous influx of immigrants from the "old" world. To work the statistics in a different way, in 1775 one out of every eight hundred Americans was a Methodist; by 1812 it was one out of every thirty-six.[10] That, despite – or in part because of – congregational behaviour that Anglican missionary Charles Woodmason described thus: "Gang[s] of frantic Lunatics broke out of Bedlam.... One on his knees in a Posture of Prayer – Others singing – some howling – These Ranting – Those Crying – Others dancing, Skipping, Laughing and rejoicing."[11] Wigger comments, "While early Methodism cannot be reduced to enthusiasm, neither can it be understood without it."[12]

The Tension

A blessed season of revival may require greater

---

[10] John H. Wigger, "Taking Heaven By Storm" *Journal of the Early Republic*, 14 (Summer 1994), p.167.
[11] *Ibid*, p.177.
[12] *Ibid*, p.191.

discernment than any other period of church life. The "Toronto Blessing" is not about the manifestations – but rather, it is about the Father blessing His children. Having firmly established that central declaration, we have to be quick to say that the "Toronto Blessing" cannot be understood without the manifestations. Eivion Evans traces this same tension at work in the Welsh revival of 1904-5:

> Oh, what a scene it was! The whole place was in apparent confusion, some praying aloud, others confessing their sins, many of the heathen in agony appealing to God for pardon, some even fainted, so great was the power. It was a pleasure to hear some of the older Christians praising God and shouting, 'The Church now lives! The Church now lives!'
>
> Throughout the progress of the work the leaders showed a remarkable willingness to follow the lead of the Spirit, even though the sight of physical prostrations, dancing, and wild excitement would have been previously repugnant to them.[13]

Brynmor Jones is even more descriptive in some of the accounts he records of the same revival: "The sober, sedate Calvinistic congregation that gathered in Mount

[13] Eivion Evans, *The Welsh Revival of 1904-5*. Bridgend: Evangelical Press of Wales, 1989, p.156.

Seion that morning received a shock." It was not their own pastor leading, but Evan Roberts and his "worship team."

> The divine assaults of the Eternal Spirit were seen striking down men like corpses all over the floor.... [N]ot a few were frightened at the sights they saw.... I know of a man of lukewarm temperament, and of a cold and precise philosophical turn of mind, on the spur of the moment being set ablaze like a bonfire; and all who saw him going wild, clamouring, and bounding like a hart back and forth from the ground floor to the gallery, and from seat to seat through the chapel, thinking that he had for certain taken leave of his senses.... His opinion to this day is that the Sprit of the Lord in a supernatural way was moving him from the narrow circle of his reason, his understanding, and his knowledge, to the wide world of the spiritual.[14]

* * *

"Do you approve or disapprove of the meetings on the whole?"

Sixty years earlier, revival swept through much of

[14] Brynmor Jones, *Op. cit.*, p.159-60.

Scotland. One of its leaders was WC Burns, of Kilsyth Church. On September 1, 1841, he wrote a letter in which he unguardedly names the discredit and animosity brought against him; the balance of the letter is a description of the work of grace in which he was privileged to play a part:

Perhaps you have heard of the wonderful things which the great God has been doing for us in Scotland. The servants of Satan have reviled God's blessed work; and I wish to tell you something of the truth about it. You know that may people come from the church the same way as they went to it; the Word does not touch their consciences, and they remain under the power of sin and Satan, of death and hell. This used to be very much the way among us until lately; but the God of love has visited us, and poured out His life-giving Spirit upon the dead souls of men. In some places you might see the solemn sight of hundreds weeping for their sins, and seeking to give up their hearts to Jesus. And, ah, what a sweet change has taken place on many! The high looks of the proud have been brought down; dead formalists have become living Christians; worshippers of Mammon have been changed into lovers of God; the blasphemous tongues of the profane have made to sing God's praise....[15]

Though the local pastor of Kilsyth, Burns also preached itinerantly, and along with other revival leaders, he was mightily used of God in the autumn of 1839. Through his ministry, the Lord graciously ushered in a new season of fervour and awakening in a number of parishes throughout Scotland. This was so much the case that in December, 1840, the Presbytery of Aberdeen appointed a committee to examine reports of the revival that was sweeping the area. They had "concerns," and so issued a questionnaire for their pastors to complete.

While conducting a pastor's conference in Edinburgh, I was handed a copy of this questionnaire, *"Evidence on Revivals: Answers to Queries on the Subject of The Revival of Religion in St. Peter's Parish, Dundee."* The pastor responding was Robert Murray McCheyne. I found the Presbytery's questions and McCheyne's reflections to be most interesting and engaging. McCheyne completed the questionnaire on March 26, 1841, and was commenting on the church's experience over the last nineteen months, since August of 1839. When I was given the following account, it was about the same amount of time that had transpired since January 20, 1994, and the beginning of the renewal in

[15] William C. Burns, *Revival Sermons*. Edinburgh: The Banner of Truth Trust, 1980, p.9.

Toronto. There is over a hundred and fifty year spread between McCheyne's time and ours. So much has changed in a century and a half; yet there is a certain timelessness to the theological and pastoral issues raised by an outpouring of God's Spirit. The following is an abbreviated version of the questionnaire McCheyne was asked to answer. Such extended consideration is given to his responses because it provides considerable insight into how a previous "renewal" unfolded, such that historians speak of the "Scottish Revival of Religion." The concerns and questions, and the reflections and resources brought to bear can serve us as we attempt to discern the renewing and reviving work of the Spirit in our midst, in our day.

By way of context, Robert Murray McCheyne was one of Scotland's bright lights, a leading, respected and honoured pastor. He knew enough Hebrew to be able to converse with European Jews. He read the Greek classics for pleasure, and to keep his journal private, he made his entries in Latin. For the record, McCheyne and his fellow Presbyterians maintained the five classic points of Calvinism: total depravity, unconditional election, limited atonement, irresistible grace, and the perseverance of the saints.

These are the questions to which McCheyne was to respond:

1. "Have revivals taken place in your parish or district; and if so, to what extent, and by what instrumentality and means?"

2, 3 and 4. These raised issues of the "previous character and habits" of those involved. Have any abandoned their evil practices? (Drunkenness and neglect of family duties and public ordinances are specifically named.) Have any become "remarkable for their diligence in the use of the means of grace?" Has there been recognizable life-change?

5. "Has the conduct of these parties been "consistent; and how long has it lasted?"

6. The same questions (2-5) are asked, but corporately considered, not only for the local church, but the surrounding region.

7. "Were there any public manifestations of physical excitement, as in sobs, groans, cries, screams?"

8. "Did any of the parties throw themselves into unusual postures?"

9. "Were there any who fainted, fell into convulsions, or were ill in any other respects?" (It seems that there is some bias against the manifestations!)

10. "How late have you ever known revival meetings to last?" (Understood in the context of a strong Calvinist work ethic, this question makes more sense than it might otherwise. Is it likely to be God at work if those "revived" are up so late the night before that they're no good for work come the next morning?)

11. "Do you approve or disapprove of the meetings upon the whole? In either case, have the goodness to state why."

12. "Was any death occasioned, or said to be

occasioned, by overexcitement, in any such case? If so, state the circumstances, insofar as you know them." (The issue here is the attempt to bring clarity to exaggerated and distorted reports of the meetings.)

13. "State any other circumstances connected with revivals in your parish or district, which, though not involved in the foregoing queries, may tend to throw light upon the subject."

Mr. McCheyne answers as follows:

1. On revival: "It is my decided and solemn conviction that a very remarkable and glorious work of God, in the conversion of sinners and edifying of saints, has taken place in this parish and neighbourhood." He had begun his ministry in that parish in November 1836, four years earlier, and while there had been "evident blessing from on high in many instances," "there was no visible movement among the people until August 1839, when the Word of God came with such power to the hearts and consciences of the people, and their thirst for hearing it became so intense, that the evening classes in the schoolroom were changed into densely crowded congregations in the church" that gathered together for worship almost every night for four months. Thirty-nine "house groups" also began during this period, five of which were "conducted and attended entirely by little children." He names several visiting ministers who assisted in the work; McCheyne says, "I have good reason for believing that they were eminently countenanced by God in their labours."

"As to the extent of this work of God, I believe it is impossible to speak decidedly." He notes that people came from "all quarters of the town," from "all ranks and denominations of people." "I am deeply persuaded, the number of those who have received saving benefit is greater than anyone will know till the judgement day."

2-3. On life-change: "... Not a few have become new creatures." "Many, again, who were before nominal Christians are now living ones." Some, were radically converted from "paths of open sin." He names the power of a credible witness: "I often think, when conversing with some of these, that the change they have undergone might be enough to convince an atheist that there is a God, or an infidel that there is a Saviour."

4. On numbers: McCheyne recognizes that it's impossible to keep an exact account of all "awakening or conversion; and there are many of which the minister may never hear." He does state that in the autumn of 1839, not fewer than 600 to 700 "came to converse with the ministers about their souls."

5. On conduct and consistency: "Many who came under concern for their souls have gone back to the world." But in that "remarkable season in 1839, there were very few persons who attended the meetings without being more or less affected. But many allowed it to slip past them without being saved ... and alas! There are some among us, whose very looks remind you of that awful warning, 'Quench not the Spirit.'"

McCheyne knows of only two who "have openly

given the lie to their profession." But "many there are among us, who are filled with light and peace and are examples to believers in all things."

McCheyne describes extra communion services held as the "happiest and holiest" he ever attended. The entire day was spent in thanksgiving and a special offering was generously given, and sent to missions.[16]

6. On regional influence: McCheyne reflects that, sadly, the majority in Dundee remain unmoved, "still sunk in deep apathy in regard to spiritual things, or are running on greedily in open sin."

But, he names special favour from the Lord to establish nineteen Sabbath schools, all of which were well taught and well attended. Previously, these had been impossible to institute. (The issue of special favour will feature prominently in future considerations.)

7-9. On public manifestations: "There were many seasons of remarkable solemnity, when the house of God became literally a 'Bochim, a place of weepers.' Those who have present at the meetings, I believe, never will forget them.... I have seen the preaching of the Word attended with so much power, and eternal things brought so near, that the feelings of the people could not be restrained." He says there have been times of "awful and breathless stillness," "half-suppressed sighs," "many bathed in tears," "a loud sobbing." Some,

[16] The themes of gratitude, generosity and mission are recurrent in true revival.

"cried aloud, as if pierced through with a dart." All of that, *during the preaching*.

But it's not *just* tears of repentance that characterized the meetings.

McCheyne continues, "I have seen persons so overcome, that they could not walk or stand alone. I have known cases in which believers have been similarly affected through the fullness of their joy...." He concludes his comments of the manifestations with a call for discernment: "I am far from believing that these signs always issue in conversion, or that the Spirit of God does not often work in a more quiet manner. Sometimes, I believe, He comes like the pouring rain; sometimes like the gentle dew."

10-11. How late do the revival meetings go, and do you approve?

(Note McCheyne's response to naming things "revival.") "None of the ministers who have been engaged in the work of God here have ever used the name *revival* meeting; nor do they approve of its use. We are told in the Acts that the apostles preached and taught the gospel daily; yet their meetings are never called revival meetings."

As to the meetings, they usually went to ten o'clock. Sometimes, there was such a move of the Spirit, they had to stay longer, so many sought prayer – sometimes till midnight.

"On such occasions I have longed that all the ministers in Scotland were present, that they might learn more deeply what the true end of our ministry is.... The feelings that fill my soul are those of the most solemn awe, the deepest compassion for afflicted souls, and an unutterable sense of the hardness of my own heart. I do entirely and solemnly approve of such meetings,... and it is my earnest prayer that we may yet see greater things than these in all parts of Scotland."

12. Any deaths? Yes, but the report on the thing was maliciously distorted. "A groundless calumny."

13. There was space on the questionnaire for further reflections. As many of us have done in the midst of this current outpouring, McCheyne studied previous revivals, in order to understand what he was experiencing. He reviewed the historical records of other revivals in Scotland, and the Great Awakening in America and concluded: "The outpouring of the Holy Spirit ... was attended by the very same appearances as the work in our own day. Indeed, so completely do they seem to agree, both in their nature and the circumstances that attended them, I have not heard a single objection brought against the work of God now which was not urged against in former times, and has not been most scripturally and triumphantly removed by President Edwards in his invaluable *Thoughts Concerning the Present Revival, and the ways in which it is to be acknowledged and promoted.*"

McCheyne then quotes Edwards: "And certainly we must throw by all talk of conversion and Christian experience; and not only so, but we must throw by our

Bibles, and give up revealed religion, if this be not in general the work of God."[17]

Exponential Consequences

As God renews and revives His people in these special seasons of grace, it is as if the wind of His Spirit ripples the pond. The effects of His powerful presence are felt in ever widening circles of influence, often beginning with pastoral leadership, then throughout local congregations, and then beyond the walls of the church.

As to how this is felt out on the edge, there is a telling anecdote of a conversation that takes place between the circuit riding Methodist preacher, Fransis Asbury, and a young man, roughly two hundred and twenty years ago. The young man approached Asbury and said, "Heard you were at the Methodist meeting." "Sure was," came the reply. "Any shouting?" "Some." "Why do Methodists shout?" "Because they're happy." "Well," replied the young man, "I can't see how anyone could be happy in church. Whenever I go I feel like a corpse."[18]

As the dialogue song between the shouting Methodist and the Formalist made so delightfully clear, revival typically begins with the reviving of the preacher. As

[17]*Memories of McCheyne, II: Messages and Miscellaneous Papers.* Andrew Bonar, Moody Press, Chicago, n.d., pgs. 221-231.
[18] Charles Ludwig, *Fransis Asbury: God's Circuit Rider* (Milford Michigan, Mott Media, 1984), p.1.

McCheyne's reflections indicate, the next to be revived is the local church. While unsettling to many, the physical manifestations that so characteristically accompany an outpouring of God's Spirit play an important role in taking things further.

What Draws the Unsaved?

One of the ways to understand the physical manifestations that often accompany a reviving work of the Holy Spirit is that they serve as God's own advertising. To change the metaphor, they are like fisherman's bait. A bare hook in the water generates little by way of interest; what's needed is something on there that draws some attention. In the midst of all that's taking place in revival meetings, it is the physical manifestations that generate a significant amount of attention!

To look at things another way, consider the following: why did unbelievers come out to hear Wesley preach? Because they woke up one morning, and figured they had better go get saved? At least as Wesley records in his *Journal*, some were drawn for other reasons:

> "*Curiosity* led [a young woman from London] to hear a sermon, which cut her to the heart. One standing by, observed how she was affected, and took occasion to talk with her." The two corresponded by letter; the first was

told, 'Christ is ready to receive you: Now is the day of salvation.' Quickened, she responded, 'It is! It is! Christ is mine!' and was filled with joy unspeakable."[19]

The phrase, "they came, either to hear or see" recurs in Wesley's daily entries, as in the following account:

Edward Farles had been an hearer for many years, but was never convinced of sin. Hearing that there was much roaring and crying at the prayer-meetings, he came to hear and see for himself. That evening many cried to God for mercy. He said himself he wished it was all real; and went away more prejudiced than before, especially against the roarers and criers, as he called them. But soon after he got home, he was struck to the ground, so distressed that he was convulsed all over. His family fearing that he would die, sent for some of the praying people. For some hours he seemed to be every moment on the point of expiring ... but, about four in the morning, God in a moment healed both soul and body. Ever since he has adorned the Gospel.[20]

---

[19] John Wesley, *Journals*. Grand Rapids, Michigan: Baker Book House, 1984. February 17, 1772, p.453. Italics added.
[20] *Ibid.*, June 5, 1772, p.471. See also December 21, 1776, p.90.

In his classic work, *Revival,* Martyn Lloyd Jones reminds his readers that if revival broke out in the church, "the man in the street, and all his friends would come in."

Why? Quite simply: "He comes because he has suddenly heard that something strange and wonderful is happening in that church.... The man in the street is only attracted finally by power."[21]

Jones then cites Acts 2.12-13, "they were amazed and perplexed, and asked, 'What does this mean,' and others said contemptuously, 'They have been drinking!'" By way of comment, he candidly reflects on the characteristic ways in which unusual phenomena accompany a revival of religion:

> There are people, who dismiss, and denounce, the whole notion of revival because of these phenomena, and therefore when they are exhorted to pray for revival, they say, 'Most certainly not. We do not want that sort of thing. We are not interested in that kind of experience.' And, thus, without realizing it, they are often guilty of quenching the Spirit.[22]

Brynmor Jones, in *Voices From the Welsh Revival*

---

[21] Martyn Lloyd Jones, *Revival*. Wheaton: Crossway Books, 1994, pgs. 61-2.
[22] *Ibid.*, p.136.

traces similar dynamics, when he comments that

> the strange coldness and passiveness of the [visiting] ministers, content to remain mere observers, robbed them of the blessing.... The powerful emotional upheavals of this kind did not go down well with all the ministers and church leaders.... [Nevertheless], people came for very mixed reasons and even the most distinguished visitors confessed to new experiences. Many came originally to watch events but were consequently caught up in them.... No one had seen meetings of this kind before and it is little wonder that the many visitors were fascinated. One can share the feelings of that aged man who called out, 'I came three thousand miles to this meeting, but I would go round the world to see such as this.'
>
> The consequence [of the revival within] the Church is that it is made attractive to the world. People cannot help going to church or chapel now. Sensible men, though they may be unsympathetic, talk respectfully about the Church of Christ today. Moreover the Church is aggressive. Awakened itself to its own needs, it has at the same time been awakened to the needs of the unconverted and unregenerate world outside. It can be said of

the Church of Wales ... that great grace is upon all. There is the grace of love and compassion.[23]

Open Doors

In terms of a characteristic process of revival, what seems to take place is that first and foremost, the Lord graciously renews, refreshes, and releases leadership; their influence, in turn, brings transformation to local congregations. The renewed, even revived church moves outside of herself with new passion, vision, confidence, boldness and authority to share the love of Jesus. Combined with a sensed "season of favour" initiated by the Lord Himself, spiritual doors swing wide open as never before.

This has repeatedly been the case in our present experience. On May 24, 1995, seven of us were invited to be the featured guests of the Phil Donahue Show, one of the leading North American day-time TV talk shows.[24] Characteristically, Donahue has not been particularly interested in the Church of Jesus Christ. The few times he has had Christian leaders on the show, he has been caustic, accusatory and fault-finding. The only reason Donahue was interested in us at all was because of the reports of hysterical laughter. The physical manifestations continue to prove to be

---

[23] Brynmor Jones, *Op. cit.*, pgs. 79, 116, 114, 155, 200.
[24] The show aired September 19, 1995.

provocative; so much so that he extended to us the invitation to talk about our experience on prime-time television.

We spent a great deal of time praying about the invitation, and felt that the Lord had opened a significant door for us, so we accepted. We were able to go with wonderful freedom, in part, because we realized that the Lord had called us to be His witnesses, not His lawyers. We would share what we had experienced of the power of our Heavenly Father's love and grace, and leave things at that.

With incredulity, Donahue read from various headlines: *The Toronto Star*: "Laughing all the way to Heaven." *Florida Today*: "Floored by God." Another, "Church that has them rolling in the aisles." *Christian Week*: "Toronto Blessing garnering worldwide attention." Another: "Holy high jinx: thousands flock to church that's just for laughs." It was the manifestations, especially the laughter, that held Donahue's interest, and that, because it was so very far outside of his own experience in church. As he turned to my wife, the first person he interviewed, he asked, "Janis Chevreau, you believe this is God manifesting Himself through the people in attendance. Do I understand you?"

For fifty-one minutes, the seven of us got to talk about the grace of God, the love of the Lord Jesus Christ, and the powerful presence of the Holy Spirit, before a viewing audience of thirteen million people. That's the largest congregation any of us had ever preached to! And because of very favourable audience response, the show has been re-televised repeatedly.

The New Life team of the Toronto Airport Christian Fellowship knows when the show has re-aired, because when they ask the newly saved why they have come forward for prayer, the answer comes: "I saw you guys on the Donahue show, and I had to see if it was for real."

One man from Michigan, for instance, watched the re-run in June of 1996. He was so moved by what he saw of the supernatural power of God, he said to his wife, "I just have to go to that church this Sunday." He made a four-hour drive to Toronto, and responded to the altar call at the end of the Sunday morning service. With tears streaming down his face, he surrendered his life to Jesus.[25]

Urban Rebirth

As the wind of the Spirit continues to blow, the pond's ripples move further and further out. Not only are individuals converted; the grace of God redeems and revives whole communities.

In May 1995, Vineyard pastor and overseer Steve Phillips, was invited to speak at Bethesda Full Gospel Church in Buffalo, New York. This is an inner city, predominantly black congregation of about 900

[25] As reported by John Arnott, *Spread the Fire*, August 1996, vol.2, #4, p.2.

members led by Pastor Michael Badger. Many from the church had been attending meetings at the Toronto Airport Vineyard since the early days of the renewal. Steve has preached several times at TACF, and without knowing it, had prayed for a number of this congregation while ministering in Toronto.

When he was at Bethesda, one young man named Melvin Taylor asked him if he remembered the prophetic words he had given to him in Toronto. The word Steve had spoken to Melvin was that God was going to use him to raise up gangs of people to go through the city doing spiritual drive-bys, "shooting" prayers of blessing at those walking and standing on the streets. Further, the Lord would be sending him to the street corners of the nations to proclaim His Word, such that revival would come through the inner cities.

Melvin had received a similar word prior to Steve's from Grace Lee, of Woman's Aglow. Upon hearing it again, Melvin decided it was time to get on with it!

What Melvin did not know was that the youth pastor, Kenny Williams, had received a word that he was to cancel the weekly youth meetings, and begin weekly "drive by" prayer attacks in a very crime-ridden neighbourhood nearby. At first he thought this could not be God. "The church will never put up with this!" he reasoned. But the leading would not go away, so he arrived at church one night ready to announce this new plan to the youth group when he noticed the choir practising on stage. Immediately, he felt God say, "Go tell the choir director that he is supposed to cancel practice and take the choir in the lead cars like the tribe of Judah leading Israel around Jericho!" Kenny had little faith for a favourable response. He was surprised, therefore, when the choir director simply said, "Alright, I will."

For several weeks they drove around the neighbourhood, singing praises and praying as they passed gang members on the street. Several times they saw the Spirit of God move significantly as people would come over to the cars to talk with them. On one occasion a young man wept as he accepted Christ. He then displayed the gun he had under his coat – he said that he was on his way to kill someone.

During all this time, Melvin was unaware of Kenny's street worship and prayer activity. On his own, he was planning to do a tent meeting in a neighbourhood that was known for its gunfire, prostitution and heavy drug traffic. Without any money except his pastor's support, Melvin ordered the tent and wrote cheques for all of the necessary equipment and began the "Possessing the Land" meetings that ran from July 17th until September 3rd, forty-nine days in total. On the third day of the crusade, one of the cheques bounced.

The person who sold Melvin the tent was very upset, and threatened to repossess his merchandise. Melvin assured him that the funds were forthcoming. At the conclusion of their business negotiations, Melvin got on his knees. By the time he'd finished praying, calls of support and financial assistance began coming from numerous sources.

The meetings were blessed by a powerful outpouring of the Father's presence. Some four hundred people responded to the Lord's call. The churches from the city began to support the meetings.[26]

From the time the tent was set up, there were no reports of shooting or murders in the ten block, three avenue perimeter that was sealed off by the prayer walks and the drive-by blessings. A year before, fifty murders were committed in that area. In a television interview, the police commissioner stated that "for some reason that he was not sure of," the neighbourhood's crime rate had dropped 33% compared to the previous year. There had been significant drug busts; key drug dealers had been arrested, and many crack houses were shut down.

When Melvin returned to the neighbourhood recently, local shopkeepers and community people came to express their gratitude and support for what Melvin had started the year before. Many of them reported that the neighbourhood was a completely different place, and that their business profits were significantly increased, up from the previous year. They were also quick to add that their stores had not been robbed since the meetings.

I asked Steve Phillips to reflect on his experience at

[26] Melvin can be reached by fax at 716-884-3595.

Bethesda. He commented:

> In Ezekiel 36:33, God says, "On that day I will
> cleanse you from all your iniquities, I will also
> enable you to dwell in the cities and the ruins
> will be rebuilt." Perhaps we presumptuously
> believe that we know what it takes to build a
> society and live together. It's just possible that
> the destruction of our cities is an outgrowth of
> that presumption. It may be that we will not
> see the problems of crime, violence and drugs
> solved until we, in humility, ask the Father to
> cleanse us and "enable us" to dwell in the
> cities. I believe Michael Badger's congregation
> is a shining example of this model of spiritual,
> urban rebirth and revival.

* * *

Monday is the only night of the week when there is
no evening meeting at the Toronto Airport Christian
Fellowship. Consequently, many out-of-town visitors
rent a car and drive around Lake Ontario to Niagara
Falls. Those who do so in the month of May are awed,
not only by the grandeur of the mighty Niagara, but also
the acres and acres of blossoming fruit trees along the
highway.

Blossoms are a good way of thinking about the
physical manifestations and the wonderful work that the

Spirit of God is doing in our midst. The fruit trees on the Niagara Escarpment are not planted and cared for in order to produce blossoms, as beautiful as they are. It is as St. Augustine commented on John 15.6: *Aut vitus, aut ignis.* Freely translated, it's "fruit, or firewood." May's blossoms are at best signals, pointers, the "manifestations," of a larger, longer dynamic at work. What is taking place is an "impartation" of sap that, under proper conditions, yields September's fruit-bearing.

There are many people who come to relish the beauty of the blossoms, in and of themselves. But there are many more who come months later to pick their own. Many more still eat of the harvest, without ever seeing the blossoms that "advertised" the wonderful season of new growth that had been initiated months earlier.

The balance of *Share The Fire* is a consideration of the evangelistic fruit that our Lord purposes us to bear as we abide in Him and His words dwell in us.[27]

---

[27] John 15.7.

CHAPTER THREE

CHURCH GROWTH, RENEWAL, AND GRACE BASED EVANGELISM:

A Confession

* * *

You and we belong to Christ, guaranteed as His and anointed, and it is all God's doing; it is God also who has set His seal upon us and, as a pledge of what is to come, has given the Spirit to dwell in our hearts.
2 Corinthians 1.21-2

* * *

My doctoral thesis was titled *A Pastoral Explication of John Calvin's Instruction on Private Prayer.* It represented the culmination of a six year study of sixteen centuries of God's renewing, reviving work in His Church. Upon its completion, I needed to catch up with what was currently happening and so devoted myself to the study of Church growth literature, a very different world from the historical and theological research I had done previously. Nevertheless, I found the field engaging, and read widely.[1] Following many of

---

[1] *A partial list of titles is indicative of some of the themes considered: Where Do We Go From Here; Activating the Passive Church; Unleashing the Church; Sharpening the Focus of the Church;*

the footnotes to their sources, I read some of the current business literature as complement.[2]

I also spent my study leaves at various church growth conferences. Among other places, I went to Willowcreek Community Church, in North Barrington, Chicago. From the senior pastor, Bill Hybels, I "caught" some of their evangelistic passion for those whom they have affectionately called "unchurched Harry and Mary."

All of this study clarified my thinking, sharpened my vision, and taught me a lot about evangelism, leadership and the ministry of the local church. It was the resource pool from which we drew as we articulated the mission philosophy and mandate for the church we were attempting to plant in the fall of 1993.

Without diminishing or dishonouring the value of things learned in formal study, eclectic reading, and time spent at Willowcreek and other Church growth

---

Outgrowing the Ingrown Church; The Church on Purpose; Prepare Your Church for the Future; Growing a Healthy Church; Twelve Keys to an Effective Church; Marketing the Church; Leading Your Church to Growth; Leading and Managing Your Church; Mastering Church Management; Management of Ministry; Managing the Non-Profit Organization.

[2] *Teaching the Elephant to Dance; Thriving on Chaos; Running Through Walls; Barbarians to Bureaucrats; Leaders; Becoming a Leader; The Visionary Leader; Leadership and the One Minute Manager; The Art of Leadership; Servant Leadership; Principle-Centered Leadership; Why Leaders Can't Lead; The Leadership Secrets of Attila the Hun.*

conferences, the Toronto Blessing has made it clear to me that it is not so much what is taught, or caught, that makes the transformative difference in a church's life and mission; it is what is *given*.

Reaching the Unchurched

In the very early '90s, one of my friends relayed the following story to me. At the time, he was the senior pastor of a "significant" university church. After their annual report was reviewed, he was asked, "Pastor, have I missed something – there doesn't seem to be an evangelism committee here at this church; is that under the mandate of the missions commission?" He responded, "No ... evangelism is really the mandate of the entire church...." There followed a pregnant pause, the "oh-oh ..." kind. *"Evangelism is really the mandate of the entire church...."*

My pastor friend confessed ZERO conversion growth that particular year. I felt as chagrined as he did. Our net conversion growth for that year was 2.3%, but those two couples were our "harvest" after six years of ministry.

At the time, my pastor friend and I were working through the rather depressing book, *Fragmented Gods: The Poverty and Potential of Religion in Canada.* In it, Bibby cites the growth studies he conducted of evangelistic churches in Calgary, a Canadian city demographically similar to the one in which I was living at the time. In findings he titled, "The Circulation of the

Saints," Bibby stated that the net conversion growth for the surveyed churches was 1.9%.[3] Given the fact that I had been preaching , I felt, passionately, "The Church exists for those who are not yet a part of it," and that "we in Christ are God's missionary people," and that, indeed, "evangelism is the mandate of the entire church," it was small comfort that we were ahead of the Calgary average by .4%. For *that* particular year. We were pathetically below average if previous years were factored into the equation.

So convinced was I of the primacy of evangelism that I resigned the traditional church I had been pastoring and devoted myself to planting a church where I would be working with those similarly devoted to an uncompromised commitment to reaching the unchurched. In Oakville, the community to which we moved, well over 90% of the people we surveyed believed in God. We had to hold a rather open definition – some believed their *cat* was God – nevertheless, over 90% believed in something more than themselves, something more than the material world. They believed in something of transcendence. However, only 4% of Oakville were in church on a Sunday. One could rightly draw a quick conclusion: "God, yes; church, no."

On the home front, the book *Cinderella* was one of my daughter's favourites. We read and re-read it together. One night, as I was looking out the window,

---

[3] Reginald Bibby. Irwin Publishing, Toronto, 1987, p.30.

the glass slipper scene clarified what I knew intuitively. If traditional churches were meeting the needs of the 90% who believed in God, they would be in church. If things were the right size and shape and style, it would be a wonderful "fit." But by their not being in church, it was an indication that for all sorts of folks, the traditional "glass slipper" did not fit.

Our mission mandate became crystal clear: we were "in business" (I was reading a lot of business management material) because we recognized that there were a whole lot of folk in Oakville who would never fit the glass slipper, as beautiful and precious and formative as that slipper was for many. We were "segmenting the market," knowing that there are a whole lot of people who have been raised wearing Nike running shoes, folks who would NEVER fit the slipper.

Organized to Death

With a well-researched, carefully crafted and illustrated mission philosophy in hand, we knew what our vision was; we had clear goals and guiding principles; we had a magnificent five-year plan.

Our core mission value was declared simply enough: we were committed to "intentional relational evangelism." Strategically, we taught the maxim: "Figure out what you love doing, and go do it with the unchurched." To model it, my co-pastor, Kim, and I went to the local yacht club and asked if there were any skippers looking for crew. A few days later we received a call from Bill.[4] He had just bought a new boat, and wanted to race Tuesday nights. Were we interested? Were we interested?!

For the next several Tuesdays, we had an exhilarating time aboard a 36-footer, with seven other unchurched guys. Kim and I were doing a great job of "intentionally relating." We'd race for an hour and a half and then spend three hours shooting the breeze. During that time, we heard non-stop bravado, conquest, and testosterone. After five weeks, the skipper finally got round to Kim and me and asked, "What do you guys do for a living?" When we answered, "We're pastors," their faces went blank as they re-wound the tapes of the previous five weeks' conversations....

I developed a good relationship with Bill, and we got along swimmingly as long as we related as one entrepreneur to another. But any time I tried to shift the conversation to "spiritual things," the conversation ran aground and became forced. That was painfully the case when I tried the "Bill, if you were to die tonight ..." question.

Let the reader understand: Bill is the most successful businessman I know. He is the most intelligent, synthetic, global, trans-national thinker I have ever been privileged to meet. One could very easily, and correctly, conclude that he has the world by the tail, and that he owns a significant part of it – tax-free.

---

[4] His name has been changed.

"Bill, if you were to die tonight...." He sent non-verbals that indicated that he thought the question was beneath both our dignity. He answered, "I'm not going to. Die. Tonight." And that was the end of that. We changed the subject of conversation to spinnakers and depth-sounders.

Ancient Scripts

Along with the Church growth literature I had read, there was a side-line study: burn-out. It has little to do with the length of time one works: we can find ourselves burned-out working 30 hours a week. Burn-out is the malaise that leaves us miserable day after day, week after week, month after tedious month. Physiologically, its symptoms include difficulty in sleeping, weight loss or gain, headaches, backaches, and intestinal problems. Emotionally, burn-out is characterized by chronic tiredness and irritability, low-grade to desperate depression and nagging boredom.

At the forefront is a crisis of expectations. There rises up a systemic disappointment as expectations exceed experience. "The best laid plans of mice and men...." In the pastorate, most have high hopes to see the church grow; with that hope, there are diverse and contradicting congregational expectations as to the conduct of a pastor's ministry, such that no pastor can possibly meet them all. Regardless of what he or she does, it will not be right in somebody's estimation, and they'll more than likely say so – to someone else.

Especially as a church planter, I found myself attempting to function with both a chronic shortage of resources and a pervasive sense of inadequacy. Together, they acted catalytically to generate full-blown despair, and with it, a fatigue, and sense of frustration, even failure. Things kept erupting into not-so-occasional outbursts of rage. When those fire-storms had settled, the climate was one of a deep loneliness.

Much of the literature suggests solutions to burn-out that encourage one to manage time more effectively. Again, there are some great books that are invaluable resources.[5] When surveyed and distilled, the common denominator of the time management literature is strategic goal setting and prioritization. Thoreau put the issue dynamically: "For every thousand hacking at the leaves of evil, there is one hacking at the roots." Instead of attending to symptoms, address the causes. The thing was, I *had* a carefully crafted personal *and* corporate mission statement. I understood that it was "value driven work" that yielded the highest dividends; the "driven" bit, however, I always found unsettling. It seemed to stir some deeply imbedded scripts down in wherever scripts are embedded. I could almost see the clipped comments, in red, on the side bars of my childhood report cards: "Can do better." "Guy fails to apply himself."

[5] *The One Minute Manger; The Time Trap; Time Power; Seven Habits of Highly Effective People* and *First Things First.*

Especially in the context of the church plant, my performance orientation was in full bloom. I was suffering from acute "results anxiety," especially with respect to evangelism. Like a hungry, commission-driven salesman, I was trying to close the deal; the response I was getting was, "Just browsing; killing time." Even if it was eternally.

Illusory Reprieve

In the burn-out literature, some of the things that came highly recommended were spiritual retreats, keeping a journal, and regular recreational activity. Come freeze-up and the end of the year's sailing, what I did to "recreate" was devote an hour of my Tuesday evenings to the TV show *McGyver*. Every week, McGyver would get himself into an impossible situation and, against incredible odds, extricate himself using whatever he could find at hand, along with his ever-present roll of duct-tape and his Swiss Army knife. My favourite episode saw him deep in Central America; his mission: to rescue a captured American agent. She was being held prisoner by subversive guerrillas. He sneaks in and finds her, gets her out of prison and, with a tarpaulin and bamboo, makes a hang-glider. While machine guns are blazing and bombs going off, the two of them leap from a cliff, and soar to safety.

McGyver's ingenuity and tenacity served me well in the midst of my burn-out. Not only was it a great mental break; it was highly inspirational. No matter how desperate the situation, he would never give up. When I would run aground doing whatever it was I was trying to do, I would look out the window and ask myself, "What would McGyver do in this situation?"

The trouble was, my gummy roll of duct-tape and fancy Swiss Army knife were not enough to see me through. The "hang-glider" that I built did not fly – we jumped off the cliff, and my "intentional relational evangelism" and the church plant we so carefully and creatively constructed not only did not carry us; it crashed pitifully, and we barely escaped the wreckage.

Reflecting on things at length, I realized something that I never read in the literature. Burn-out is rooted in bitterness. Any time we commit ourselves to a cause, however noble it may be, we will end up frustrated. The reason is that we do not have the resources necessary to see a noble cause through to its fulfilment. Over time, this frustration becomes bitterness, and this bitterness poisons us to the core. I found it a sobering coincidence that ten days before we went to our first meeting at the Toronto Airport Vineyard, February 1st, 1994, my kidneys were on the verge of failure. I very nearly died of systemic septicaemia, the medical name for full-blown blood poisoning. Upon my doctor's examination, I had no externally infected sight. He was quite puzzled, as there was no determinable source to the infection that raged within my body. I knew better.

I had become so frustrated because I knew that I did not have what I needed to see our church plant "cause" through to fulfilment. Again, our carefully crafted mission philosophy stated that we were committed to "intentional relational evangelism." Mine was forced and driven. While I truly enjoyed the friendships with the unchurched that I was making, my faith-sharing was not motivated by a heart-compassion for my friends who did not yet know how much God loved them. Rather, if I am honest enough, it was fuelled by my need to succeed, to demonstrate to the core group, the support churches, my denominational executives, other clergy colleagues, and any one else who was even mildly interested, that my ministry was viable. I needed my new friends' conversions to show in hard numbers that I was able to evangelize and grow a church.

Our mission goal was "conversion growth of 60%, to be assessed semi-annually." But my co-worker and I had to develop a way of ducking the "How big's your church?" competition. Our answer: "Something under a thousand." In actual fact, our weekly attendance was somewhere in the twenties, more or less. Numbers alone do not tell the whole tale: our growth curve was taking a nose-dive. We were losing core members fast.

That's why McGyver was so recreationally distracting. While I was exploring the landscape of failure, I would live vicariously his success vistas. If only I, too, could snoop around in the cupboard, or attic, or laundry room; in the workshop, the garden house, the junk yard – and come up with whatever was needed. Oh, to be like McGyver – no matter what the situation, he was infinitely resourceful, and resourced.

It was such a short reprieve. Come 9.00 PM every Tuesday night, I would again be face to face with my existential bankruptcy. For all my carefully strategized, prioritized, and consecrated intentions, things were just about over. I was mad at myself, and mad at those who were supposed to be working with me. I was mad at God for not seeing His end through. And the Church growth gurus' inspirations were not motivating any longer: "The greatest barriers to church planting are in the mind. Once we make up our mind to do it, it can be done."[6] I *had* made up my mind; the thing was, a hand had appeared, and I could read the handwriting on the wall: *Mene mene tekel upharsin* – "Weighed in the balance and found wanting."[7]

Up by our Bootstraps?

I should have known better. Motivated by a strong (stubborn) will, I had unwittingly embraced a pragmatic Pelagianism. Pelagius was a priest who lived in the latter part of the fourth century and early decades of the fifth. He taught a self-confidence, specifically with respect to personal holiness. Within his lifetime, his teachings were condemned as heresy, for they were essentially salvation by works, an overstatement of human freedom and the power of choice. As the

[6] C. Peter Wagner, *Church Planting for a Greater Harvest*. Regal Books: Ventura Cal., 1990, p.27.
[7] Daniel 5.25-28.

unrecognized father of "self-actualization," he gave no recognition to human limitations.

One of the Doctors of the Church, Augustine of Hippo, countered Pelagius. In a treatise titled *On Faith, Hope, and Love,* he refutes Pelagianism at length. With optimistically gritted teeth, Pelagius argued, "My liberty is such that I can do all things." Augustine responds, "Your freedom accomplishes nothing without God. It depends on Him in everything, for everything. The only thing you have that's all your own is your sin. *That* you can manage all by yourself, without God's help."[8] Augustine understood Pelagian self-determination as the very root of sin – and the very denial of salvation in Christ: rather than our attempts to *ascend* to spiritual heights, God's grace *descends* to us in Christ. Augustine frequently quoted 1 Corinthians 1.30: "By God's act you are in Christ Jesus; God has made Him our righteousness, our holiness, our liberation." Again he says, "The Son of God came that ... He might enable us who were the sons of men to become the sons of God ... that we might become partakers of His own nature."

Working from Romans 9.16, "God's promise ... does not depend on human will or effort, but on God's mercy," Augustine continues:

The whole work belongs to God, who both

---

[8] See Augustine's *Enchiridion,* Ch.30, p.247, Nicene and Post-Nicene Fathers, III. Ed. Philip Schaff, Hendrickson Pub., 1994.

makes the will of man righteous, and thus prepares it for assistance, and assists it when it is prepared.... [His mercy] goes before the unwilling to make him willing; it follows him willing, that he may not will in vain.[9]

Augustine's prayers, even more than his treatises, so convey the contrast to a self-willed determinism:

Let me know You, You who know me; let me know You, as I am known. You are the strength of my soul; enter into it, and prepare it for Yourself, that You may have and hold it without 'spot or wrinkle.' This is my hope ... and in this hope do I rejoice....
Too late did I love You, O Beauty, so ancient, and yet so new! Too late did I love You! For behold, You were within, and I without, and there did I seek You; I unlovely, rushed heedlessly among the things of beauty You have made. You were with me, but I was not with You.... You called, and cried aloud, and forced open my deafness. You did gleam and shine, and chase away my blindness. You shed Your fragrance about me; I drew breath and now I pant after You. I tasted, and now I hunger and thirst for You. You burned in me

[9] *Ibid.*, Ch.32, p.248.

the fire of Your love, and I am inflamed with love of Your peace.[10]

Re-reading Augustine's *Confessions* called forth my own. Exercising all the will I could muster, I had embraced a "pro-active self-directedness" with the best of intentions. Committed to church growth and evangelism, I had "made up my mind" to go out and do it. As I am a continuous learner, I submitted to those who were "doing it," to the point of giving serious consideration to the counsel one of my Church growth mentors who said, "In terms of leading the church, my MBA (Master of Business Administration) is of greater value than my MDiv (Master of Divinity).

What I encountered at the Toronto Airport Vineyard was a counterpoint, a complete pendulum swing: I found grace. Better, *grace found me.*

And that is the Gospel of Jesus Christ. As I have travelled around the world these last two and a half years and addressed pastors and leaders from the broadest of denominational cross-sections, there is this common denominator to the testimonies: the vast majority have embraced a cause of one form or another. They are devoting their time, energy and resources to seeing a particular end through to fulfilment, with or without a five-year plan. If candid, and most are, they

---

[10] Augustine, *Confessions*, XX.1 and 27, Nicene and Post-Nicene Fathers, I. Ed. Philip Schaff, Hendrickson Pub., 1994, pgs. 142 and 152. The syntax has been modernized for ease of reading.

declare openly that they are facing a measure of burn-out and personal bankruptcy.

Coming to a "Catch the Fire" conference is, for many of them, like calling the emergency services: during the call to prayer ministry, someone hears their cry for help. Many have been suffering a spiritual angina for years; some pastors have come with very serious "chest" pains. And some have had the electro-shock paddles put to them – with a powerful jolt, life surges into their bodies and spirits, and they feel as if they have been given another ten years.

One of the things I have discovered is that just as with heart attack victims, so it is with spiritually "zapped" and revived people. There are some who nearly immediately return to their old, driven ways. I more than understand. That is the way I am naturally inclined. I love to control, direct, and lead; those who know and love me call it my inclination to "strive, drive, and connive." I thoroughly enjoyed the energy, the synergy, the adrenaline rush that comes from "closing the deal," be it in terms of making proposals to denominational executives, or securing funding, or property, or recruiting staff. I love the creativity and independent achievement of the entrepreneur. In fact, an "entrepreneurial spirit" was near the top of the list for "Characteristics of Successful Church Planters," and on my profile test, it was my highest score. I had appropriated the key leadership principle that states "leadership takes responsibility." I interpreted this to mean that if anything was going to happen, it was up to me to MAKE it happen.

Past tense. Understood. There are some heart attack victims who undergo a radical life change. Getting "zapped" comes as an "awakening." It is the wake-up call of wake-up calls. There is a complete re-evaluation of what is left of life, and a revision of priorities and commitments, a re-statement of purpose and life orientation. Characteristically, the drivenness is transformed into gratitude. There is the recognition that life *could* have been over, finished, done. But then there has come "re-vival." Thereafter, every day, is a gift; a bonus. Some folks quite literally start stopping and smelling the roses. I know I do.

Leadership does take responsibility, but responsibility is the "ability to respond." I had been trying to initiate so much, I had *way* outstepped myself. In terms of Church growth, and especially evangelism, this has such profound consequences. The next two chapters ground a revived life in the initiative that *God* takes. With that foundation firmly established, we can then consider the response that is appropriately ours in Christ.

CHAPTER FOUR

GRACED TO BLESS:

A Study in the Acts of the Apostles

May the Lord direct your hearts into the love of God and the steadfastness of Christ. 2 Thessalonians 3.5

* * *

The "Toronto Blessing" has been provocative. While there is much that should stay on the margins, there are other dynamics that cause us to think, yet again, about the core fundamentals of faith. Grace is one of those essentials. Over the past months, I have been pulling down book after book, that my understanding of the grace of God may ever enlarge and deepen.

I began by reviewing some of my theological training: at seminary, our systematics text was Paul Tillich's three volumes. "The term grace qualifies all relations between God and man in such a way that they are freely inaugurated by God and in no way dependent on anything the creature does or desires."[1] Tillich's definition is something short of gripping; his

---

[1] Paul Tillich, *Systematic Theology*, vol.I. University of Chicago Press, 1967, p.285.

abstractions at best stretched one's mind. His philosophical theology rarely touched my heart.

Karl Barth, in his monumental *Church Dogmatics*, is also germanicly abstract: in Volume II, on *The Doctrine of God*, he defines grace as God's "unconditional, transcendent condescension."

> Grace is the distinctive mode of God's being in
> so far as it seeks and creates fellowship by its
> own free inclination and favor, unconditioned
> by any merit or claim in the beloved, but also
> unhindered by any unworthiness or opposition
> in the latter – able, one the contrary, to
> overcome all unworthiness and opposition.[2]

I was about to move on when I looked up the following reference that took on new meaning in light of so much that has characterized the Toronto Blessing: "God's glory is His overflowing, self-communicating joy. By its very nature it is that which gives joy.... And where it is really recognized, it is recognized in this quality, with its peculiar power and characteristic of giving pleasure, awakening desire, and creating enjoyment."[3] One wonders what Barth would have made of the "holy laughter"!

[2] Karl Barth, *Church Dogmatics*, vol.II. Edinburgh, T.T. Clarke, 1957, p.353.
[3] *Ibid.*, p.653.

Roughly a century earlier, the preacher-theologian, C.H. Spurgeon wrote of grace in concrete terms:

> Faith occupies the position of a channel or conduit pipe. Grace is the fountain and the stream.... Our life is found in 'looking to Jesus" (Hebrews 12.2), not in looking to our own faith. By faith all things become possible to us. Yet, the power is not in the faith but in God in whom faith relies.... See, then, that the weakness of your faith will not destroy you. A trembling hand may receive a golden gift.... The power lies in the grace of God, and not in our faith.... Think more of Him to whom you look than of the look itself. You must look away even from your own looking and see nothing but Jesus and the grace of God revealed in Him.[4]

Three hundred years earlier still, the pastor-theologian, John Calvin, reflected on Psalm 59.10, "My God, in His unfailing love, will go before me ..." and Psalm 23.6 "His mercy will follow me...." In his comments, Calvin quoted Augustine: "Grace anticipates unwilling man that he may will; it follows him willing that he may not will in vain." Calvin closed with Bernard of Clairvaux's prayer: "Draw me,

---

[4] C.H. Spurgeon, *All of Grace*. Whitaker House, 1981, p.45.

however unwilling, to make me willing; draw me, slow-footed, to make me run."[5]

Forty years earlier, Martin Luther wrote of grace in his *Preface to the Acts of the Apostles*: "It should be noted that by this book St. Luke teaches ... that the true and chief article of Christian doctrine is this: we must be justified alone by faith in Jesus Christ, without any contribution from the law or help from our works.... It all adds up to one thing: we must come into grace."[6]

The Baptism From Above

The following is a study of the Acts of the Apostles, and its two controlling themes. The first of these is the outpouring of the Spirit on the first disciples; the second is the spread of Christian faith through the conversion and baptism of new believers. A close study of these twin dynamics is especially germane in this current outpouring as it brings revival and empowers for evangelism, for the controlling message throughout the Book of Acts is *all is grace*.

Though "The Acts of the Apostles" is the name of the book, its author, Luke, makes it clear at the outset that it is the companion volume to the Gospel, and as such, it is the continuing record of what is now the second period, or phase of Jesus' work. Because the Gospel of John is sandwiched in between the two volumes of

[5] John Calvin, *Institutes of the Christian Religion*, II.3.12, trans. F.L. Battles. Philadelphia: Westminster Press, 1960, p.306.
[6] Luther's Works, *Op. cit.*, p.363.

Luke's work, we may miss just how closely the Acts of the Apostles flows directly from his account of the Gospel of Jesus Christ. The opening verse of Acts makes this connection abundantly clear: "In the first part of my work, Theophilus (literally "God-lover"), I gave an account of all that Jesus did and taught from the beginning until the day when he was taken up to heaven...."

In Acts, what Jesus commenced in the flesh as recorded in the Gospel, He now continues in His new humanity, the Church, through the leadership of the apostles. Luke makes it clear that there is a pivotal moment in this transition: his account of the Gospel ends with the resurrection and ascension, thereby bringing to an end the story of Jesus. The Acts of the Apostles marks a new beginning, commencing with a re-telling of the Lord's ascension. But this time it is connected, not with what has gone before, namely the resurrection, but with what follows, Pentecost. In other words, the ascension "finishes" the story of Jesus, and at the same time, marks the "beginning" of the story of His Church.

In a sermon titled, "The Spirit Giveth Life," the Danish theologian, Soren Kierkegaard preached on these opening verses from Acts:

> There sit twelve men, all of them belonging to that class of society which we call the common people. They had seen Him whom they adored

74

as God, their Lord and Master, crucified; as never before could it be said of anyone even in the remotest, it can be said of them that they had seen everything lost. It is true, He thereupon went triumphantly to heaven – but in this way also He is lost to them: and now they sit and wait for the Spirit to be imparted to them, so that thus,... these twelve men are to transform the world – and that on the most terrible terms, against its will. Truly, here the understanding is brought to a standstill![7]

If our understanding has not been "brought to a standstill" in this fresh move of the Spirit, let us at least proceed slowly as we reconsider familiar texts. In Acts 1.4 and 8, Luke provides a summary of the last encounter the disciples had with the resurrected Jesus: "While He was in their company He directed them not to leave Jerusalem. 'You must wait,' He said, 'for the gift promised by the Father, of which I told you.... You will receive power when the Holy Spirit comes upon you; and you will bear witness for me in Jerusalem, and throughout all Judea and Samaria, and even in the farthest corners of the earth.' "

Before we proceed, it serves to note Luke's purpose for his account of the Gospel: he is giving an account of

[7] Soren Kierkegaard, *For Self-Examination*, trans. Walter Lowrie. Princeton University Press, 1941, p.105.

"all that Jesus did and taught from the beginning until the day when He was taken up to heaven, after giving instructions to the apostles whom He had chosen." We so quickly skim over these introductory lines that serve as summary; few readers will have noted, for instance, that the rendering of Acts 1.2 is missing a phrase that is key to Luke's understanding, not only of the ministry of Jesus, but the ministry of the disciples as they live as the Lord's witnesses. The instruction that Jesus gave to His disciples was "*through* the Holy Spirit." Luke here indicates how Jesus conducted His ministry. He does so, not on His own, but, as the Gospel makes it clear, "armed with the power of the Holy Spirit."[8]

After His ascension, Jesus is no longer physically, bodily present to His followers. But through them, He continues His ministry, through the Holy Spirit. To make this essential dynamic crystal clear, Luke will not have the Spirit's work in the Church understood to be separate, independent, or dissociated from Jesus. In terms of the giving and receiving of the Spirit, and the evangelism and mission that is the fruit of the impartation, we must closely examine the key texts in Acts.

Acts 1.4-5

These opening directives are foremost to our considerations: "He told them not to leave Jerusalem.

[8] Luke 4.14.

'You must wait,' He said, 'for the gift promised by the Father.... Within the next few days you will be baptized with the Holy Spirit.'" This text makes it clear that in terms of the coming of the Spirit, there are absolutely no conditions imposed.

The first disciples were told, not that they had to remain in Jerusalem, but that they were not to depart, they were not to move away – they were not to get scattered. Secondly, they were to wait – but that is not where the emphasis lies in the text. Rather, this instruction is more pastoral than it is spatial. The instruction to "remain" and to "wait" is more of an admonition against discouragement: "It's not over yet!" There is a sense of an anticipatory directive – something "big" was about to happen, and it was the Lord's intention that none of them miss out.

It was nothing to which they had to apply themselves, however, for the focus of these verses makes it clear that the Holy Spirit is given as gift. The baptism is not "the opportunity," "responsibility," "quest," or even "privilege" of the believer, but "the promise of the Father" (v.4). Here an implicit contrast has been struck, for in Judaism knowing the "promise" was dependent on the keeping of the Law. But this gave rise to what has been noted as "the uncertainty of Judaism." The rabbis reflected on this tension:

> "God keeps to what He says, but am I among those who will inherit the promises if I do not

keep the Law?" "David said: Lord of the
world, I may confidently hold fast to Thee ...
that Thou wilt reward the righteous in the
future; *but* I do not know whether my portion
will be among them or not."[9]

There is no "but" in Acts 1.4, for there are no
conditions that must be met before the gift is given. This
is a fundamental Gospel essential that cannot be
overstated, especially when in some revival circles there
is counsel to "press in" and "take hold" of the blessing
of God. Some even cite that obscure text in Matthew
11.12, that "the Kingdom of Heaven has been subjected
to violence, and violent men are taking it by force."
Desperate believers are encouraged in a militant,
forceful seizing of the appointed hour. But all of that is
our works, not God's grace. It misses the Gospel by a
covenant, for in the Rabbinic tradition it was clearly
taught that there was an inseparable link between the
Holy Spirit and a life which is obedient to God. Outside
of Christ,

the gift of the Spirit is especially viewed as a
reward for a righteous life. Possession of the
Spirit is in the first instance the result of a
righteous life, not the basis of such a life....

[9] *Theological Dictionary of the New Testament*, ed. G. Kittel. Grand
Rapids: Eerdmans Pub. Co., vol.II, p.580.

Rabbi Nehemiah concludes: 'He who undertakes a commandment in faith, is *worthy* that the Holy Spirit rests upon him.' Rabbi Acha says, 'He who studies [Torah] with the intention of doing it, *deserves* the gift of the Holy Spirit.' 'He who sacrifices himself for Israel will receive the wages of honour, greatness, and the Holy Spirit.'[10]

The Apostle Paul meets this dynamic head-on, contrasting Law and promise, human effort and God's free gift of grace. It is the very point of his central theological argument in Romans 4.13-16:

> "It was not through Law that Abraham and his descendants were given the promise.... If the heirs are those who hold by the law, then faith becomes pointless and the promise goes for nothing.... The promise was made on the ground of faith in order that it might be a matter of sheer grace...."

The Law and grace are polar opposites; the promise is no longer promise if it has anything to do with the Law. If the promise is something to be attained or earned, it is no longer gift. "If the inheritance is by legal right, then it is not by promise; but it *was* by promise

---

[10] *Ibid.,* vol. VI, p. 383. Emphasis added.

that God bestowed it as a free gift on Abraham."[11]

The Ground on Which We Stand

The four major Spirit passages in the Book of Acts are foundational texts from which we understand and live out the grace of our life in Christ, regardless of our subjective experiences or physical manifestations of His Spirit's presence and power.

One of the greatest pastoral challenges in the midst of this gracious outpouring is raised by those who feel they've "missed out," that they "haven't received anything," that they've been "passed by." A close study of Acts 1.4-8, the pre-Pentecost announcements; 2.1-39, the account of Pentecost and Peter's first sermon; 8.4-20, the conversion, baptism and subsequent impartation of the Spirit in Samaria; and Chapter 10, especially verses 45 and 46/11.17, the conversion and Spirit baptism of the Caesarean Cornelius and his household serve well in laying foundational groundwork for all that God is doing in this season.

In each passage there is an essential modifier that qualifies or characterizes what is taking place: the reference is either to *epaggelian tou pneumatos tou hagiou,* or *dorean tou hagiou pneumatos*, the "promise of the Holy Spirit" or the "gift of the Holy Spirit," received from God, through faith in Jesus Christ. Either modifier makes it clear that the Spirit is never achieved

---

[11] Galatians 3.18.

or obtained through any human effort.

Even the time frame that is named in Acts 1.5 declares grace: the promise will come "within the next few days," "soon," without any connection to the disciples' readiness or preparedness. Further study of the phrase "you will be baptized," makes this point even more emphatically. The grammatical voice of the promised baptism is passive (*baptisthesesthe*). The passive voice means that one is acted upon. If an active verb form were to have been used, the meaning would imply the subject's action: "baptize yourselves," or, "get baptized." The passive means just the opposite: the baptism of the Spirit is not the result of the disciples' initiative, but of the Father's purposed will. This passivity on the part of the apostles is similarly declared in the final word in Chapter 2 verse 2: "where they were sitting...." They were not required to be praying, or fasting, or yielding, or tithing – just sitting. Luke is carefully relaying the fact that no activity on anyone's part can diminish the coming of the Spirit as an unearned gift.

This is mirrored in the final promise of the resurrected Jesus in Luke's Gospel: "Wait here until you are clothed (*endusesthe*) with power from on high" (24:49). The verb tense and mood here is aorist subjunctive – the sense is that of submitting as another helps you into your jacket. Again, receiving "the gift promised" is not a human or even spiritual achievement, for the text makes it clear that the gift's source is "from on high," "from heaven," (2.2) above and beyond anyone's reach or grasp. The only one "making things happen" is the Father.

Grammatically, it would have been possible to have used the subjunctive voice for the promise in Acts 1.5: the subjunctive literally means to join or add to something. The subjunctive verb form is used to express condition, contingency, possibility. It would then be rendered as "You *may*, you *might*, you *can be* baptized with the Holy Spirit." But such a declaration would send some into a never-ending spiral of soul-searching introspection – "Am I worthy? Do I deserve such a gift? Do I have enough faith?" Alternatively, the imperative could have been used: it would then take on the sense of something commanded, "You *must* be baptized." And then, there would be work for us to do: the linear thinkers among us would soon generate "five essential steps" that unfailingly guarantee the baptism.

The good news is that the promise is simple future indicative. The indicative is used to assert fact: "You *will be* baptized." There are absolutely no demands made or conditions named; there is nothing to be added in terms of human effort; nor is there any suggested uncertainty as to the promise's fulfilment.

Notice too that Jesus did not promise the Spirit only to "some," to those who were spiritually prepared, those who were humble enough, or hungry enough, or broken, to those who were empty enough to be filled. While the spiritual dispositions of humility, hunger, brokenness and emptiness serve us well, they are not prerequisites for receiving the gift of the Holy Spirit. The promise of the Father is given to every believer present, without exception or qualification, every time – from the one hundred and twenty at Pentecost, to the twelve believers at Ephesus. Nowhere in Acts does a select group of believers receive the Holy Spirit while others are excluded or "passed over." Concluding his comments on these opening verses in Acts, Bruner puts the heart of the proclamation succinctly: "The Holy Spirit comes as inclusively as He does unconditionally. Both belong to His character as gift."[12]

Acts 1.6-8

End-time theology holds a certain unbalanced attraction for some. In Acts 1:6-8, Jesus re-focuses the apostles' curiosity and speculations about the coming of the future Kingdom and puts it squarely on *mission and evangelism*. That, and not eschatology, will characterize their ministry. Further, it is made clear that this is not something that the disciples do on their own, at their own initiative, in their own strength. In 1.8 the phrase, "you will receive power," is again in the simple future tense rather than the subjunctive or imperative. It is a sovereign declaration, and neither a possibility nor a command. Further, perhaps even the preposition used

[12] Frederick Dale Bruner, *A Theology of the Holy Spirit*. London: Hodder and Stoughton, 1970, p.159.

as the Holy Spirit comes "upon" them is declarative of the sovereign, gracious givenness of the Spirit. He does not come from "within" them; the empowerment they need is not to be called forth from emotional or even spiritual longings or disciplines on their part.

This sovereign impartation of power has express purpose, for Jesus declares: "you shall be My witnesses." In the following testimonies show how the Lord used two people in this very way.

In July 1995, Vineyard pastor Steve Phillips was preaching at the renewal services hosted at the Tabernacle Church in Melbourne Florida. His theme was prophetic evangelism. Tami describes the consequences this teaching had on her.

I was privileged one night to be in a renewal service where Steve Phillips was sharing. I was so stirred as I listened to him share about how it's like our Heavenly Father has a family business and allows us as His children the privilege of working alongside Him. He also shared that when Jesus was on earth He only did what He heard the Father saying, and that's how we should be living our Christian lives.

That night as I left the Tabernacle, I realized that my car needed gas. It was late at night and I wasn't happy about stopping for gas, but I felt the Lord telling me to stop at a place called "Smiley's". As I pulled in, I noticed a large group of teens hanging out by the pay phones. The situation concerned me because there seemed to be only one girl in the midst of several boys. As I stood pumping my gas, I prayed for them.

When I was done, I walked into the store to pay my bill. The boy working behind the counter looked to be in his early 20's. I must have had a look of concern on my face, because he asked, "What's wrong?" I told him I had something on my mind, that I was concerned about the situation outside. He said, "Oh, you don't have to be afraid of them." I told him I wasn't afraid, only concerned.

I went over to the side of the store to buy myself a drink. It was then that I felt the Lord telling me to ask this boy if he went to church anywhere. As I approached the counter I said to him, "You're probably going to think I'm strange for asking this, but do you go to church anywhere?" To my surprise he said yes and that he used to go to the Tabernacle Church. I couldn't believe it; I told him I had just come from there. He said he had gone there a long time ago and that he had been a part of the "Overcomer's Ministry."

He then proceeded to talk about Bob Warner who was and still is head of this ministry. The young man seemed to be fond of Bob. I then felt the Lord saying that I should ask if I could pray with him. I did, and he said yes, and extended his hand to me. I told him I knew he was at work and if anyone came in I would understand that he would need to wait on them. He told me that his name was Joe. We prayed for perhaps a minute, and then a customer walked in. I know that it must have looked pretty funny to that man as he entered the store and saw the two of us holding hands! The Lord does have a sense of humour!

I said goodbye to Joe, and assured him that this was God at work, not me; that I didn't normally go around to gas stations at 11:30 at night asking people where they go to church so I could pray for them. I told him that God had some family business to take care of that night, and that He was giving me the awesome opportunity to be a part of it. As I got in my car to leave, I noticed that the car in front of me had stalled. There were four large young men in the car, and I asked the Lord if He wanted me to ask them if they needed help. He said no, and I sensed then that it would have somehow been dangerous for me. I remembered Steve Phillips' words that we were only to do what we hear the Father saying. And then I realized that we're not meant to minister to everyone, but only those the Lord is calling us to.

Another Tabernacle member, Bob Deacon, takes over the story. Bob is a well-ordered engineer whose ministry has previously been that of teaching. He has served both as an elder, and in other leadership capacities. He has been profoundly reconstructed in this season of renewal, and this particular night, he was called to give away what he had so freely received.

After receiving a very pointed and accurate word from the Lord through a lady who barely knew me, I decided on the way home from the Tab to try some of the stuff that Steve Phillips had been talking about.

I stopped for gas at midnight and asked, "Lord, how are You at work here?" The store attendant was the only one around, and I got a very strong impression that he would be someone Bob Warner would have ministered to. I went into the store after pumping my gas and found myself saying to the young man behind the counter, "Bob Warner says 'Hi'." I was amazed at myself for saying such a statement; the guy behind the counter was more amazed. After a long pause, he asked, "You mean, Bob Warner of the Tab?" I nodded. Another long pause, and then, "How does he know I'm here?"

I was wondering the same thing myself! I started asking a few questions, when the young man interrupted and said that someone else had been in the store a half hour earlier and was talking about the Tab, saying that he needed to go back there. He had a look of astonishment on his face.

He then figured that I must have a mobile phone, and must have talked with Tami after she left the gas station. He had so convinced himself that she and I must have talked, that he went out to check my car for a phone. When he saw that I didn't have one, he settled into the fact that much more was going on than he was comfortable realizing. He asked me what time the "Masses" were at the Tab. I told him, and shared with him something of the grace of God.

It was certainly evident that the Father was working on that guy, that night; I'll never forget the blessing I received as I played my part as the Lord's witness. It was easy!!!

Acts 2.1-4

The "ease" of a life of grace is mirrored in the timing of the outpouring of the Spirit, "when the day of Pentecost had come."[13] Rather than the fulfilling of conditions or spiritual requirements, the outpouring of the Spirit is dependent only on the sovereign timing of God. Again, the Spirit's "source" is named: "from heaven...." He comes "suddenly." There is nothing of the apostles' readiness, preparedness, or worthiness that plays any part in their reception of the Spirit.

This is the case when the gift of tongues is given. *Each* of the gathered receives the gift, and *all* are filled with the Holy Spirit. In fact, when all of the Spirit passages in Acts are reviewed, nowhere is there a record of one or several persons being passed over with the full gift of the Spirit because they are somehow unworthy or unprepared.

Acts 2.14-36

The heart of Pentecost is not found primarily in the inner, deeper spiritual experience of the first disciples, nor even in the outpouring of the Spirit, but in the

13 Acts 2.1.

ability, freedom and authority to preach Jesus Christ. This causes a shift in most of our thinking, for typically when we think, "Pentecost," we think "Spirit." But the very purpose for the gift of "other tongues" is the ability to tell other "people groups" about the great things that God has done in His Son Jesus. Here in Acts 2, tongues are given, as it were, in order that the cursedness of Genesis 11 might be reversed. The confusion that concludes the Babel story is turned so as to bring about the oneness God purposes in Christ. Commenting on this passage, Calvin states: "God furnishes the apostles with the diversity of tongues now, that He may bring and call home, into a blessed unity, men which wander here and there.... Wherein appeared the manifest goodness of God, because a plague and punishment of man's pride was turned into a matter of blessing."[14] The redemptive purposes of God in Christ are clearly demonstrated in the very content of Peter's preaching, for what Peter preaches is not the Spirit, but Jesus. From Joel's prophecy, and the pouring out of the Spirit on *all* flesh, Peter's preaching crescendos with verse 21, "Whoever calls on the name of the Lord shall be saved." The purpose of the eschatological outpouring of the Spirit is in the universal promise of salvation, to "repent and be baptized in the name of Jesus the Messiah for the forgiveness of sins." Upon repentance and baptism,

---

[14] John Calvin, *Commentary on the Acts of the Apostles,* vol.I., Grand Rapids: Baker Book House, 1993, p.75.

Peter assures his first hearers that *they* will receive the gift of the Holy Spirit; "for the promise is to you, and to your children, and to all who are far away, everyone whom the Lord our God may call."[15] Once again *gift* and *promise* are named, as are God's sovereign initiating and choosing. Neither is the end or focus of Peter's sermon, but rather is the consequence or result of receiving forgiveness in the name of Jesus.

In our day, there are some wonderful testimonies as to how the Lord our God is yet calling those who are "far away," and bringing release as "sins are forgiven." Having been to one particular church several times, I've had the opportunity to witness the longevity and life-change of one gloriously graced conversion.

Nicky's story was simple. He grew up knowing about religious things, for his father was the choir director in an Orthodox congregation. He prayed childhood prayers for help and blessing, and as a child, he was quite sure that "it" was true. At about the same time he became an altar-boy, he also got hooked on street drugs. By ninth grade, he was a frequent user of acid, cocaine, speed, and mescaline. Alone in the sanctuary, he robbed the congregational offering boxes, finding them to be a ready source of funds for his drug addictions.

Fifteen years of drug related drama went by, until July 1995, when in desperation, he called his cousin, Mark.

[15] Acts 2.39.

After a great deal of confusion, it slowly became clear that Nicky was trying to explain that his girlfriend had seven or eight distinct personalities – which were a few more than Nicky could cope with. Mark promised that he would help, but only if Nicky promised to come to "the meetings." Nicky had been through rehab before; he thought he was headed for another try at a twelve step program.

The "meetings" that Mark had in mind, however, were the renewal meetings hosted by the Tabernacle, in Melbourne Florida. Nicky was brought to the Catch the Fire Conference in August. Lying out on the carpet the first night, the Lord graciously set Nicky free. He testifies that he was completely delivered of his addictions, not just from the drugs, but alcohol and cigarettes as well. No one prayed specifically for any of this; rather, simply "More, Lord." Having experienced the power of His Spirit, it was easy to explain to Nicky the power of salvation in Jesus' name.

The Spirit filled Nicky to overflowing and, as Mark tells it, "the other stuff washed out." Night after night Nicky came, finishing up on the carpet, flat on his back, "looking straight into his Father's eyes."

At the end of the conference he returned to his home. His answering machine was full of old messages from old friends – his return calls were "new messages" from a new friend with a new heart.

A year later, Nicky is still free of his addictions, and growing in the Lord. His testimony has so profoundly influenced his girlfriend that in spite of her brother's recent AIDS related death, she now knows of her Heavenly Father's unfailing love.

Acts 8.4-17

Back in the Book of Acts, the disciple Philip was one of those who went about preaching itinerantly. The apostles in Jerusalem heard of his ministry: the Samaritans had "accepted the Word of God." However, there was an anomaly: though baptized into the name of Jesus, they had not received the Holy Spirit. Bible scholars have long recognized that this is a problematic situation when compared with other texts in Scripture. In Romans 8.9, for instance, Paul makes the point explicitly that "if a man does not possess the Spirit of Christ, he is no Christian." Given such clear declaration, there is a glaring incongruity in the Samaritans' salvation experience.

In working towards an understanding of the situation, it is important to note here that the remedy for the absence of the Holy Spirit is not focused on the Samaritans. The problem is not with them; nor is it with Philip and an incomplete or flawed evangelistic message. No blame is attached to anyone mentioned. In fact there is no record of further instruction being required here in Samaria; Luke does not suggest that in this regard anything more needed to be learnt. The remedy is simply prayer and the laying on of hands. While we might wish that many of the details in Acts 8 were clearer, this much is certain: as it was at Pentecost, so it is subsequently – the impartation of the Spirit is gift, unearned, undeserved, and unconditional.

The situation in Samaria, however, *is* an hermeneutical puzzle. If the absence of the Spirit was not due to any human error in the proclamation of the Gospel, why did the Samaritans not receive the "gift" as others had before them? While scholars have a field day in their interpretations of this text, few fail to recognize that Samaria was the Church's first decisive step out of and beyond Judaism, and the immediate area around Jerusalem. As such, it marked a most significant moment in the life of the early Church – relations with the Samaritans stirred deep-seated religious and racial prejudices. In other words, Samaria was the first mission outpost, the first time that the Gospel had moved cross-culturally, out beyond Jerusalem and her resident Jews.

The stalled gift of the Spirit in this unusual situation anticipates the truth that Peter fully realizes when the Spirit falls on Cornelius and his household in Acts 10: "I now understand how true it is that God has no favourites."[16] The Samaritans were *not* outside of God's favour. In terms of mission history and the expansion of the Church one understands this passage as signalling God's intentional withholding of the gift of His Spirit until the apostles should see His presence and power

[16] Acts 10.34.

manifested with their own eyes. Further, the coming of the Spirit on the Samaritans is sovereignly delayed until the apostles are themselves the instruments – the filling of the Spirit comes through the laying on of *their* hands. Then and only then do the Samaritans receive the Spirit. Now fully convinced that God's favour and blessing in Christ was breaking down racial and cultural barriers, Peter and John have no reservations in bringing the good news to "many of the Samaritan villages" on their way back to Jerusalem.

Acts 8.18-24

These verses about Simon Magus and his quest for more of the Spirit are a telling narrative about what not to do by way of seeking for more of God's Spirit. With the other Samaritans, Simon believed in the Gospel that Philip preached and, with them, was baptized. Enamoured with the miracles that accompanied Philip's preaching, Simon followed him about constantly.[17] When Peter and John came from Jerusalem and laid hands on the Samaritans and the Spirit was imparted, Simon was so "impressed" that he offered to pay for the power, not just to receive, but to impart the Spirit as well. The sense is that he wanted to add the accompanying signs and wonders to his bag of magical tricks. He thought that the Spirit was, as it were, at the disciples' disposal.

---

[17] Acts 8.13.

Simon was willing to pay, "*dia chrematon*," to give what he himself possessed. But if he could buy what he wanted it would not be grace, for God's gift comes *dia charitios*, not *dia chrematon* – by grace, not by payment. In verse 20, Peter responds with a strong rebuke: "You thought God's gift was for sale? Your money can go with you to damnation! You have neither part nor share in this, for you are corrupt in the eyes of God. Repent of this wickedness of yours and pray the Lord to forgive you for harbouring such a thought."[18]

At first, it sounds as if Peter is over-reacting. Why was Peter so vehement? How had Simon sinned against God? In speaking of Simon's request for the Spirit, Peter uses the verb *ktasthai*, "to obtain." This is the only time in all of Acts that "obtaining" is used in connection with the reception of the Spirit. Everywhere else in Acts, the gift of the Spirit is "received," *lambanei*.[19] In this light, Peter's response can be considered appropriate, for Simon had made two serious mistakes. First, he had degraded and dishonoured the Gospel by presuming that one must pay a price for what God makes free. Second, he thought that the Spirit was theirs to bestow, as if "it" were a commodity that they possessed.

---

[18] Acts 8.20-22.
[19] Acts 1.8; 2.33; 8.17; 10.47; 19.2.

Unqualified Grace

Seven chapters later, in Acts 15:1-29, there is "fierce dissension and controversy" raging within the early Church. What has so grievously disturbed the well-being of the Church is the way in which the gift of grace is received. There were some who were teaching that circumcision was a requisite for new believers, in accordance with Mosaic law; "Judaizers" is the name Paul gives these misguided Gospel teachers.[20] Paul and Barnabas are sent up to Jerusalem and they tell the full story of the conversion of the Gentiles. Again, the debate rages: the Pharisaic believers insist that "Those Gentiles must be circumcised and told to keep the law of Moses."[21]

This is no small issue; the very future of the Gospel and the missionary enterprise of the Church is at stake. For these reasons, this "summit meeting" is well attended. When Paul and Barnabas finish speaking to the issues, Peter takes his turn and reflects on their collective experience at Pentecost. He then rehearses the substance of his first sermon. Drawing from the revelation he received through his encounter with Cornelius, he concludes his address by speaking of the Gentile conversions: "God, who can read the human heart, showed His approval by giving the Holy Spirit to them as He did to us. He made no difference between

[20] cf. Galatians Ch.3, and 6.12-16.
[21] Acts 15.5.

them and us; for He purified their hearts by faith." Then comes his forceful conclusion: "Why do you now try God's patience by laying on the shoulders of these converts a yoke which neither we nor our forefathers were able to bear? We are saved in the same way as they are: by the grace of the Lord Jesus."[22] Corroborating Peter's testimony, Barnabas and Paul again take the floor and describe the signs and wonders God worked among the Gentiles. James gets in the final word: "We should impose no irksome restrictions on those who are turning to the Lord."[23]

We Gentiles (males especially!) could easily gloss over this passionate debate over circumcision, relieved that it has little bearing on today's Church. While conformity to Mosaic law is not on the forefront of most church conflicts, the generating dynamics often are. This text represents the seedbed of legalism. The questions it raises are: What is required for full favour and status? What is expected? What must be achieved? What is the underlying "only if" – "You will only know the fullness of God if...."

The apostles together are adamant – the grace of God is unqualified. Having to submit to circumcision implies that faith is not sufficient before God; this one thing must be done in order to be fully pleasing to Him. But it's like the old story of the camel and the tent – let in

[22] Acts 15.8-11.
[23] Acts 15.19.

the nose and before long, you're out in the cold, and the camel is in where it's nice and warm. If there is *anything on our part to be done,* how do we know we have done enough? This is the very uncertainty that precipitated the Protestant Reformation: Luther asserted that with supplements, "faith and the whole Christ crash to the ground ... it is either Christ, or my own doing."

The religious exclusivism that the Judaizers were imposing was, and is, a tiny virus that eventually corrupts the whole. If anything is added in order to make faith and salvation complete, we have, even in the most innocent of conditions, the infection that leads to contamination. Cleansing, faith and the Spirit Himself are all the gracious gifts of God. Peter makes the point that all that must be achieved, God has done. Salvation is all God's work and not our own. Christ Himself lives His holiness in us; the faith which we are so often admonished to "have enough of," God grants; the Holy Spirit whom so many urgently seek, is freely given. What a relief! It is not to us to make our hearts pure, to have enough faith, or to possess the Holy Spirit; rather, it is all and only grace. God gives Himself and all His gifts, unearned, and unachieved.

By way of conclusion, Peter states: "It is by the grace of the Lord Jesus that we are saved, just as they are."[24] There is a lot of theology to be had in such a little bit of

24 Acts 15.11.

grammar: the verb tense, voice and mood of our salvation is aorist passive infinitive. That means that our salvation is complete; it is accomplished for us; and it is without end or bounds. God's grace is everything, and only where grace is everything is there good news to tell.

This passage we have been considering in Acts 15 deals with issues around salvation. But what of our spiritual disciplines and devotions as we live out our life in Christ? Without diminishing either in any way, they are, and must be, response, not initiative. This realization came home most markedly at a conference in Knoxville, Tennessee. During a pastors' question and answer session, we spent a great deal of time and energy discussing the role of intercessory prayer in renewal. There were some there who were insisting that it was a necessary and conditional precedent to revival – no prayer, no revival. We were dug in deeply; somehow Arminianism was again pitted against Calvinism. My friend Alan was with me; he has a most remarkable gift of intercession. In the midst of the disputations, he began to shake violently, as he often does, still.[25] He stood, sort of, and tried to speak: "Every revelation of the Father's heart is always a virgin birth." That rather cryptic declaration silenced all our wrangling and once we recognized the profundity of his

---

[25] See Alan's testimonies in *Catch the Fire* and *Pray With Fire*, pgs. 189-197 and 167-179 respectively.

statement, it opened the way to some of the most powerful, corporate ministry I've ever had the privilege to be part of. Walls of prejudice were shaken; significant reconciliations were initiated; a sweet spirit of worship and service came over all who were gathered, and bonds of love and commitment were formed that are having dynamic consequences in the greater Knoxville community.

We are indeed called to greater and greater Christ-likeness. We are to "go on in God," and "walk in the Spirit," and "share the Gospel." But renewal has brought grace to the forefront of my ministry assessments – I am now continuously sniffing the spiritual atmosphere, trying to discern, "Who is initiating?" "Is what is being called forth a meeting of conditions and an earning of favour, or are things as at beginning: grace alone?"

"You came to my aid even before I called upon You"

In his autobiography, *Confessions*, Augustine continuously names a dynamic of grace that we would do well to recover. Again and again, he speaks of prevenient grace. The word, *prevenient* comes from two Latin roots: *pre*, before, and *veni*, to go. God's love and mercy always precedes, anticipates, and prepares the way for our response.

I call upon You, for by inspiring my soul to long for You, You prepare it to receive You....

You came to my aid before I called upon You.
In all sorts of ways, over and over again, when
I was far from You, You coaxed me to listen
to Your voice, to turn my back on You no
more, and to call upon You for aid when, all
the time, You were calling to me Yourself.[26]

Augustine gives poetic expression to what is echoed
repeatedly in the conversion accounts detailed in Acts.
The heart of the hearer is prepared not by any activity
of his or her own, but by the electing and sovereign
Lord. The Centurion Cornelius does nothing but act on
the angelic direction given to him in a dream, sending
for and receiving God's appointed messenger, Peter,
who is likewise prepared and directed. After telling
Cornelius about Jesus, Peter concludes, "Everyone who
trusts in Him receives forgiveness of sins through His
name."[27]

Likewise, the Pharisee Saul responds to the Lord's
dramatic initiative. In Philippi, a woman named Lydia
was among those listening to Paul's preaching. In terms
of her conversion, Luke tells us that "the Lord opened
her heart to respond to what Paul said."[28] Later in that
same chapter, the Philippian jailer comes under
conviction, again because of divine intervention. He

[26] Book XIII.1, p.311.
[27] Acts 10.43.
[28] Acts 16.14.

asks, "What must I do to be saved?" What must he do? Nothing, but put his trust in the Lord Jesus. Then he will be saved.[29] Some Atheneans in Chapter 17 and some of the Corinthians in Chapter 18 hear Paul's preaching. Their conversion is simply declared: they "listened and believed."[30]

Tales of Grace

Those clipped phrases, "the Lord opened her heart to respond," and "they listened and believed" will always make me think of an evening spent in Copenhagen, Denmark. I had the privilege of preaching at renewal meetings in the city. Saturday night, after the ministry time, one of the host pastors, Johannes Fuchs, took me to the infamous red-light district. Several years earlier, as Johannes had been praying around the streets of the city, he found himself in that section of town. There the Lord spoke to him: "Johannes, it is for the sake of these people that I have called you to Copenhagen."

Four years later he received a phone call from a Pentecostal pastor who had a small cafe outreach to the drug addicts. Johannes had preached there a few times but his involvement had, up to this point, been limited. The pastor said, "Our congregation has to close the cafe because of a lack of willing workers. We have talked about you with our elders and we have agreed that if

[29] Acts 16.26, 30 and 31.
[30] Acts 17.34, and 18.8.

you will take over the leadership we will give it to you and your church – the chairs, tables, coffee machines, cups, as well as the DKK 50,000 ($12,000) in the bank."

Johannes took the work over, but he and his helpers found that very few drug addicts and prostitutes came to the cafe. The girls could not afford to leave the streets for a coffee break; once they realized this sad fact, the cafe workers went to them. In the late hours of the winter night they would go out onto the streets with thermoses of hot chocolate and coffee. They would walk up to those huddled together and ask, "Have you had a hard day? Here, warm yourself with a drink of something hot." As relationships grew, so did the off-hours visits to the cafe.

This street front ministry is appropriately called the *Klippen,* Danish for "The Rock." Johannes says their mission mandate is simple: they serve coffee, bread, and Jesus.

The business management gurus maintain that there are three keys to success: location, location, location. The *Klippen* is certainly in the right place. We arrived shortly after 12.30 in the morning and parked the car a block from the cafe on a small side-street. As we started to walk Johannes pointed and said, "Over there, a drunken sailor was murdered by a prostitute's boyfriend the previous week. They needed his money roll so they could by their drugs." We continued our tour. On the street in front of the cafe was a used syringe. Next door to the street cafe is a brothel, red neon lights and all. Immediately across the street is a heavy-duty porn video store. On the other corners are two tattoo shops, one of which is the Hell's Angels' front for their drug dealings. There are at least four sex shops within a block radius, one of which is exclusively for homosexuals. The "Men's Home" is down the street a block, providing cheap housing and meals for destitutes. Prostitutes hang about on block after block; cars cruise by and pick up girl after girl. Twice knowingly, we passed men exchanging money for drugs.

Walking with Johannes and his wife, Ann Lis, and co-workers, Lars and Ulla, was a most remarkable experience. After four years of consistent, loving service, the girls and the drug addicts know how much these folks love them. Johannes spoke by name to about fifty of his street friends in the space of our twenty minute tour. The majority that we met were heavily stoned. One women kept sniffing up the cocaine dribble in her nose. So many of those to whom I was introduced had such empty eyes, and broken bodies.

One girl was strikingly different. From half a block away, a being-redeemed prostitute shouted, "Pastor!" She came running up and gave Johannes a big hug. They introduced me as their friend, and because of her trust and honour of Johannes and his co-workers, favour was extended to me. It had happened time and again on our walk, and so surprised me. I have worked briefly in a medium security prison, and I know the agony of having to earn favour. But after chatting a bit, Rosie, the woman, gave away her cigarette, and asked if we would pray for her, right there on the street. Johannes looked at me, and asked if I would. Rosie smiled, giving her permission.

We thanked God for this precious woman, and for good friends who care so much. We thanked Jesus for being the very best of friends, for loving each of us so much, Rosie included, that He gave up His life, so that we could live. We gently prayed for the Holy Spirit to come and fill her life with the love of Christ ... she got all wobbly, and we had to hold her up.

As we turned to go, Johannes told me that since coming regularly to the *Klippen* and receiving prayer on a frequent basis, Rosie is hooking less; she recently got a job where she keeps her clothes on and has moved off the streets and into an apartment.

After our street tour, we returned to the *Klippen*. Sitting in the simple surroundings, Johannes showed me a few of the transcribed testimonies of some of the converts now working with those still on the streets. Michael, for instance, was a heroin addict who was invited to go out for pizza with some of the *Klippen* workers. While Johannes said grace, Michael saw a strong, bright light, and a person who stretched out His hands towards him, saying, "Follow Me, and I will set you free." A profound peace came over Michael and his drug buzz was instantly gone. He remembers, "Jesus

had met me, and I knew that I had to make a choice."
Johannes was sitting beside him and Michael quietly
pulled on his arm and told him to call the rehabilitation
centre.

This is Michael's testimony after seven months of
medical treatment and prayer ministry, Bible study and
friendship with other believers: "I am a new creation!
Jesus has set me free! God has put in my heart a love for
the people I used to live among. I want to tell them
about the way out of their drug addictions and their
misery. The fire of God has cleansed my heart and given
me a hunger to serve Him."

There on the bulletin board, along with "before and
after" photographs, was the story of another delivered
heroin addict, Per, who is also now one of the workers
at the *Klippen*. He had used hashish for 18 years, and
heroin, pain killers and tranquilizers for the last 10. Per
had gone through many rehabilitation programs,
unsuccessfully. In 1993, he nearly died from his drug
abuse.

Initially, Per came to the cafe only for the free coffee
and bread. When the staff would start to tell him about
Jesus, he would say, "Must you? – go away, leave me
alone." Without apology, they would reply, "Jesus is
your only hope." Over time, his heart was softened by
their love. "The life and the love that the staff radiated
– it was fantastic! I wanted to be like them. Soon I
didn't come only for their coffee and bread, but because
of their love and care." The staff at the Rock helped Per

into a rehab program. He was amazed that this time, his withdrawal from the drugs was so easy – his testimony: "I'm sure it is because they prayed for me all the time." He says, "I have never felt better in my life, and never had more peace in my mind. I thank Jesus for this!" Per is a living Psalm: "O Lord my God, I called to You for help and You healed me. O Lord, You brought me up from the grave; you spared me from going down into the pit."[31]

I will never forget how much love Johannes has for his flock, and how much they love, honour, respect and receive him. Henry, for instance, kept following us on our walk, wanting nothing from us except to be with us. In fact, no one asked for anything but prayer.

That night, down the street from the Copenhagen bus station, I saw enfleshed what it means to be "a friend of sinners and prostitutes."

Last Look

The way to new life in Christ is only and always one's response to God's initiating grace, received experientially. In the Book of Acts, there are never any conditions imposed. But those who know their Bibles well may be saying, "Hang on a moment – what about the conversion and baptism of the Ethiopian Eunuch?"[32] In terms of evangelism, there are several extremely

---

[31] Psalm 30.2-4 NIV.
[32] Acts 8.26-40.

important dynamics at work here. The first is that the one used of the Lord is not Peter, but Philip. He, unlike Peter, is not a high-profile apostle. While named as among the first disciples, he is one of the faceless hundred and twenty at Pentecost. Philip has *only* the authority and anointing of a believer in Jesus Christ. Yet it is clear that he is the one whom the Lord chose to lead this dignitary to salvation. Further, Philip does not suddenly come under conviction, and make a willed decision to do a bit of evangelism Wednesday nights. The Holy Spirit initiates and arranges the meeting with one who is divinely prepared.[33] It is also the Spirit who concludes the encounter – the Spirit "snatches Philip away."

After Philip preaches Jesus, the Ethiopian asks, "What is there to prevent me from being baptized?" Eighth century editions added the next phrase, Philip's response: "if you believe with all your heart, you may." Because it is well established as a late addition, most Bibles put this in the margins or footnotes.[34] This is not hypercritical nit-picking, but an imperative distinction: nowhere else in all of Scripture is believing with all one's heart made the condition for salvation. None of us yet believes with *all* our hearts. As we each pray, "Lord, I believe; help me in my unbelief," we rest in the knowledge that all is of grace.

---

[33] Acts 8.39.
[34] New International Version, Revised Standard Version, Jerusalem Bible, Revised English Bible etc.

* * *

The revelation of undeserved, unmerited, unearned grace spans the centuries, and brings redemption and transformation wherever and whenever it is declared with power and authority. The "glory of free grace" was one of the distinctives that marked the Welsh revival under Daniel Rowland, Howell Harris and William Williams. In April 1739, one hearer summed up the preaching: "The New Covenant is all of grace, the beginning, growth, and ending; He is the Alpha and Omega; it is all of grace, so this jealous God will have all the glory of man's salvation to be ascribed to His free grace in the face of Jesus Christ."[35]

[35] Eivion Evans, *Daniel Rowland and the Evangelical Awakening in Wales*. The Banner of Truth Trust, Edinburgh, 1985, p. 130.

CHAPTER FIVE

LEARNING FROM THE MASTER:

Grace Rediscovered

Filled with compassion, Jesus reached out His hand....
Mark 1.41

* * *

It is as if the scales have fallen off my eyes. This revelation of grace has reduced everything else to zero. I have ransacked my shelf of books on evangelism, and I now see things so very differently.

One of the early texts I read was Lewis Drummond's *Evangelism*, which maps out the "foundational guidelines on how to evangelize in a local church."[1] Drummond contrasts the traditional "come structures" of a local church – "Come to our Sunday morning program," with a basic re-orientation of ministry mandates, such that there are "go structures" in place. Logistically, he names the process: there must be the setting of goals or aims, a surveying of the surrounding community, a surveying of the organizational life of

---

[1] Lewis Drummond, *Evangelism*, Marshall, Morgan and Scott, London, 1972.

church, and a surveying of the church leadership. But as we attempted to put all of that into practice in the local church through the mid-1980s, we found that this process consumed what seemed to be an inordinate amount of time, energy and paper; we found that systemic and institutional ills were being uncovered, and while the uncivil war raged internally, it is now no surprise that precious few were being led from darkness to light.

Coleman's *The Master Plan of Evangelism* and Kennedy's *Evangelism Explosion* at least got us out into the community, but for most of us, what we found was that a lot of doors kept slamming in our faces, and we did not get around to much faith sharing.[2] Peterson's *Living Proof* was a good read back then, and seemed to seek middle ground for the established and more traditional church: "Efforts at evangelism are often either an unannounced assault on a stranger, or little more than being nice to someone."[3] The difficulty, however, was that my "evangelistic" friendships rarely went further than nice friendships. When I recently reviewed the book, I noticed why that might have been the case: Peterson subtitles his book, *Sharing the Gospel Naturally*. Flipping through the chapters, I was struck at how *unsuper*natural his evangelism seems.

[2] Robert E. Coleman, *The Master Plan of Evangelism,* Revell Co., NJ, 1978.
[3] Jim Peterson, *Living Proof*, Navpress, Colorado Springs, Colorado, 1989, p.27.

The Holy Spirit and His work is hardly mentioned at all in the book.

With grace at the forefront of this outpouring of the Spirit, we are thinking very differently about evangelism. It is not a particular approach, philosophy, or strategy for the late 1990s that we need. As Michael Green insists, "It is the Holy Spirit Who initiates evangelism, motivates for it, and empowers it. The ways of carrying it out are legion. No, it is not methods we need, but a closer walk with the Spirit of God."[4]

To that end we take up a basic principle of scholarship and "go to the source." That has us asking, "How did Jesus evangelize?" I concede that the question is somewhat awkward, but recognize the truth in the famous statement of the communications genius Marshall McLuhan: "the medium *is* the message."

When even a few of the various encounters in the Gospels are surveyed, the distinctives of grace based evangelism begin to emerge. For instance, in John 3.1-12, Jesus and Nicodemus have an extended *tête à tête*. Nicodemus is a member of the Jewish Council, and Jesus has a wonderful time with this theologian, tangling him up with several double entendres. The first is His out-of-the-blue declaration, "You must be born again." Most Bibles have a little note beside this verse, for the original Greek has two meanings: *"genaethae*

[4] Michael Green, *Evangelism Through the Local Church: A Comprehensive Guide to All Aspects of Evangelism.* Nelson Books, Nashville, 1992, p.319.

112

anothen" can be translated as either "born from above" or "born again." Before Nicodemus can get things sorted out, Jesus tells him, "You ought not to be astonished!" He then proceeds to talk about wind and Spirit, a *doubled*-double entendre, for in Greek and Hebrew, the original words *pneuma* and *ruach* mean both wind and Spirit. In English, we miss the confusion that this conversation generates: verse 8 reads "the *pneuma* blows where it will... so it is with everyone who is born from *pneumatos*."

Nicodemus is now thoroughly tangled; he asks for clarification regarding spiritual rebirth: "How is this possible?" Jesus teases him: "Is this famous teacher of Israel ignorant of such things!" One can only wonder what Scriptures Nicodemus mentally rehearsed at this challenge – Ezekiel 37 perhaps: "Can these bones live?" "Only You, Lord God, know that." "Prophesy to the *ruach* ...." Jesus keeps him reeling: "If you disbelieve Me when I talk to you about things on earth, how are you to believe if I should talk about the things of heaven?"

In terms of their theology, no one else in all the Gospels is given such a difficult time as Nicodemus.

In the following chapter, there is an extended account of the conversation Jesus had with the Samaritan woman at the well;[5] by verse 14, the discussion has moved from its opener regarding natural thirst, to living

[5]John 4.4-30.

water. In the space of five verses we read two of the quickest transitions in all of Scripture, from eternal life, to sex and promiscuity, to a rather abstract discussion about worship and liturgy. This fast change of subject meets with no objection from Jesus; rather, things are conducted with such grace that the woman heads home to her neighbours with missionary zeal: "Come and see a man who told me everything I ever did."

Four chapters later, we have an encounter with similar situational dynamics. In John 8.1-11, the woman "caught in the very act of adultery" is brought before Jesus. Where the meeting with the woman in Chapter 4 was serendipitous, this one was a set-up orchestrated by the Pharisees. Adultery hasn't changed at all in two thousand years – then, as now, it is something more than a solo engagement. If caught "in the very act," the question begs to be asked: where is this woman's lover?

Might it be that he stayed around to see the outcome of things? As it was a set-up, might it be that he was ready to get in on the stoning, and so "destroy the evidence" of his own adultery? Knowing the secrets of the heart, is it possible that when Jesus looked up after etch-e-sketching in the dust, he looked in the direction of the woman's partner and said, "That one of you who is faultless shall throw the first stone." Might it be that *he* was the first to drop his rock to the street?

Where the conversation with the Samaritan woman ends with Jesus' self-revelation, "I am the Messiah, I who am speaking to you," this encounter in John 8 ends with words of absolution: "Has no one condemned you? Nor do I. Go and sin no more." Neither response is repeated anywhere in the Gospels.

Consider another pair of similar but contrasting encounters. In John 5.1-9, Jesus seeks out the lame man at the pool of Bethesda. This man had been crippled for thirty-eight years; over and against all of his excuses, Jesus has to talk him into his healing: "Do you want to get well?" This man is the only one in all the Gospels to whom Jesus asks this question.

In Luke 5.17-26, there is another man who is also paralyzed. Where the lame man in John 5 was a victim to his circumstances, here he, or at least his friends, are pro-active in their pursuit of healing. In the midst of Jesus' sermon, they rip the roof apart, and lower him bed and all, before the preacher. Talk about pressing in! Jesus asks no questions of this man; he simply declares, "Your sins are forgiven."

Similarly, in Mark 1.23-26, the demoniac in the synagogue is rebuked, silenced, and delivered. But in Luke 8.26-39, the Geresene demoniac is asked, "What is your name?" This is the only record of Jesus asking for information from the demonic.

Another suggestive study in contrasts is found but a page apart in most of our Bibles. In Luke 19.3, we read that the tax collector, Zacchaeus was "was eager to see what Jesus looked like...." I have written in the margin of my Bible, Luke 5.27-29. There, Jesus calls another tax-collector to follow. Levi leaves all for a new Master, and throws a blow-out of a party to introduce Jesus to all his old friends. Conjecture: had Zacchaeus missed Levi's "tax collector's bash" held in honour of Jesus but heard so much about Him, that he wanted to find out for himself what all the fuss was? Might Levi have insisted, "Zacchaeus, if you ever get a chance to meet Jesus, do whatever you have to do to get near Him." And might Levi have mentioned to Jesus, "Lord, if You're ever in Jericho, look out for a short guy with a big nose... his name's Zacchaeus. He's searching right now...."

What we *do* know is that there was a most remarkable encounter: Zacchaeus gets himself out on a limb, and Jesus turns his life around: "Come down, for I must stay at your house today." Zacchaeus outdoes everyone else in the Gospels with his response: "Here and now I give half my possessions to charity; and if I have defrauded anyone, I will repay him four times over."

Across the page from the conversion story of the little man in the sycamore tree is the account found in Luke 18.18-23, the meeting of Jesus and the rich young ruler. Verse 21 sounds a most dissimilar response and conclusion: Jesus says to this man, "One thing you lack. Go, sell everything you have, and give to the poor, and you will have treasure in heaven." We read that he went away with a heavy heart; he was a man of great wealth, like Zacchaeus, but could not – correction, would not – give up his financial security for the things of eternity.

One final contrast: in Matthew 23.13-36, Jesus accosts the Pharisees and Scribes for their loveless, compassionless religiosity. There is no mincing of words: "Hypocrites! Blind guides! Blind fools! You snakes and vipers brood, how can you escape being condemned to hell!" The verse immediately following this section is a full swing of the pendulum: "Jerusalem, Jerusalem, ... how often I have longed to gather your children, as a hen gathers her brood under her wings; but you would not let Me."

* * *

Several things can be concluded from even this small sample of the individual encounters recorded in the Gospels. The first is that Jesus is not into re-runs. There is no formula to be used – John 3.3, "*You must be born again*," was not printed on a laminated card, and handed out from the street corner to everyone passing by. The Gospels record that Jesus spoke explicitly of the need for spiritual rebirth to only one person, a theologian.

Second, Jesus tunes in to each individual's life centre, their controlling passion – or pathos – and He brings compassion, clarification, and a unique response. In this, the Gospel is a 1,000-piece puzzle – its pieces – spirituality, sexuality, health, forgiveness, truth, freedom, work, money, fear, life's meaning and end.... Jesus discerned which particular piece was most needed

117

to put life together, dependent not so much on a person's presenting problems, but on the core, heart issues.

In this, there is a timelessness in the way the Lord meets us, for regardless of what we bring forward as we come before the Lord, Jesus meets us where we are, and takes us to our very depths, where His loving grace heals and restores the fractures of our hearts.

Discerning the value issues in people's lives enables us to bring a divine perspective to very nearly every discussion.

While many have mastered (with significant results), a particular opening question or formula to direct conversations through to conversion, grace based evangelism calls us beyond a particular methodology and instead invites us to be good listeners, both to the one we are with, and to the Spirit. We find ourselves praying continuously for the gift of discernment – "What do You want to do here, Lord?" "How is Your love at work in this person's life?" "What do You want to free up, release?"

Again, each Gospel encounter is situational, rather than programmatic. And Jesus is the one initiating. There are a few accounts of people forcing their way to Him, but every time, He is the one that initiates grace. Another way of seeing this is that Jesus did not take anyone for granted. The next person He met was the one on whom He had compassion.

Here, a single phrase can be pushed to the forefront:

Jesus had a divine perspective of *compassion on the next one.*[6]

In this outpouring, there has come such a precious and desperately needed softening of heart. My task orientation has yielded considerably; my self-preoccupation has turned markedly. I'm not nearly so driven. Relationally, the Spirit keeps reminding me of this phrase again and again, *"Compassion on the next one...."* And up and out of my single focus, there comes engagement and initiation: a smile, a kind word, an openness, a readiness and a willingness to go as far as the next one is willing or ready to go relationally.

For instance, I had filled my car up with gas one morning, and as I handed the attendant my credit card, she asked, "Where's our sunshine this morning?" Rather than grump about the weather with her, I grinned; "I could say, *'Standing right in front of you!'*" She certainly didn't expect that – she lit up and said, "What a great answer. I'm going to remember that!"

This sounds "soft" to some. What of eternal damnation, hellfire, judgement? What of the "urgency of the hour?" Having traced a number of encounters in the Gospels, this seems to be the *modus operandi* of Jesus; we could also take our cue from the apostles. Peter finishes his Pentecost sermon with a salvation appeal: "repent and be baptized.... save yourself from

---

[6] I am indebted to Pastor Ed Piorek of Mission Viejo Vineyard for this phrase and some of the following insights.

this crooked generation." There is a phenomenal response: three thousand are converted.

Peter does not run out and buy a tent and hire an administrator, even though "Day by day, the Lord was adding new converts to their number." In Chapter 3, Peter and John are on their way to Temple. No doubt they were talking about mission strategy and infrastructure, how to incorporate, nurture and disciple these thousands of new believers.

A beggar interrupts: "Alms for the poor?" They could have walked right by the guy, and never even see him. But something is stirred within the apostles: they stop; they "looked intently at him." Other translations read, they "looked straight at him;" they "fixed their eyes on him." What were they staring at? And why does Peter say, "Look at us"? This looking is not the usual Greek word for seeing, *eidon*, and its derivatives. This is the word used when Jesus looks at the fig tree for instance, in Matthew 21.19; it occurs 283 times in the Gospels and the Acts of the Apostles. Here in Acts 3, the apostles were "seeing" something more than just with their natural eyesight; the word is *atenisas*. From its roots, we get the English words "tension, attend, attention." This word is one of Luke's special vocabulary. He uses it twelve of the fourteen times it occurs in the Gospels and Acts. It always has a strongly intensive meaning: in Luke 4.20, after Jesus has read from Isaiah 61, "All eyes in the synagogue were fixed upon him." The word is used as Stephen "gazes intently up to heaven" in Acts 7.55. In Acts 10.4, Cornelius stares at the angel that appears in his vision; in 11.6, Peter does the same in his dream. Paul fixes his eyes on Elymus the sorcerer in 13.9; he looks intently at the cripple from Lystra in 14.9. Here, in Acts 3.4, Peter And John "see" the grace of God on this particular beggar, and miraculous healing results.

In verse 6 Peter says, "What I have I give." He says he had no silver or gold. What *did* he have? What do we have? Grace based evangelism is not an issue of our net worth or our available resources and abilities. What *we* have is not what those around us need most of all. Rather, life change comes only through a free and generous revelation of grace that makes known the loving heart of God. *Compassion on the next one.* Instead of an evangelistic drivenness, we are called to attend, listen, and love.

* * *

While at a conference in Pasadena, I had some time off, and took the opportunity to do a bit of hiking. After asking the hotel manager about places to go, I got lost on his directions. I got re-oriented with the help of a "local," and found myself at a fork in the road. I asked the Lord which way I should go and had the inclination to take the proverbial road less travelled. Seeing in the distance where I wanted to get to, I drove about trying to find an access point and, after backtracking a couple of times, it felt like at long last, I was off.

This was my chance to have a bit of Sabbath rest; it was a much needed break to enjoy the quiet of the woods while doing some super slow reading. I had brought my pocket New Testament. I read a portion of Scripture and while walking thought about how life was unfolding. I prayed both in English and in the Spirit, meditated on the Scriptures I was reading, and enjoyed the beauty of God's handiwork, the mountains and the woods through which I was hiking.

On route, I passed a man and a woman walking together. They caught up to me while I had stopped to read; I overtook them while they were resting. An hour later, I rounded a rock bluff and suddenly came upon them again, sitting in the sun, enjoying their lunch. We chatted; they passed me their carrots. We talked some more: "Where are you from?" "Toronto." "Here on business or pleasure?" "Both, actually. I love what I'm doing." "Must be nice! What do you do?" Rather than give the answer that I find often terminates conversations, "I'm a pastor," I eased into things by saying, "I'm a writer and a conference speaker." "Motivation or something?" "Something like that. Ever heard of the Toronto Blessing?"

The woman, Ellen, had, and animatedly relayed a few of the stories she had heard. "That's that laughing church, isn't it?" Her friend, Jim, looked at her and said, "Laughing *church*?" She and I began to explain. For thirty minutes, Ellen kept me engaged, asking all sorts of questions – how things began, how they had grown, and what was happening around the world. Jim was fascinated as I told stories of the power of God's love, and the radical life transformation that has come for so many people.

I felt embarrassed that I was doing most of the talking, and that the focus of the conversation was so centred on me. Several times, I tried to shift things, and asked after their work and families; Ellen especially kept wanting to hear about what God was doing in people's lives in the mid-'90s. We spoke at length about finding and being found by love, about life's meaning, about purpose, providence, and destiny.

Jim fell asleep in the sun; Ellen and I dosed off soon after he did. Fifteen minutes later, I excused myself and continued hiking. Since that meeting, I have thought a lot about Ellen and Jim. They were "the next ones," and I believe that our time together was compassion-filled. But I did not "close the deal" evangelistically. They believed in God, but didn't have a personal relationship with Jesus. I did not ask them if they would like to. And it has made me wonder.

I believe that with all the decisions about where to go, and the dithering about finding where to start hiking, there was a very real sense of a divine appointment with Jim and Ellen. Certainly their engagement reflected that. I hope and trust it was a graced encounter. Jim was still asleep when I left them. Instead of whispering "Goodbye," Ellen smiled and said, "A privilege." It made me think again that evangelism is not so much a task to complete as it is an invitation to relationship. The thing is, I had not issued them the invitation. Had I shared as much of the Gospel as they were prepared to hear? I'm not sure – I did not ask if the Lord purposed things to go further than they did. I recognize now that I had not "looked intently" as Peter and John did in Acts 3.6. I am left praying, "Lord, call the next person in to take Jim and Ellen the next step." In the grace of God, I trust that whatever Kingdom seed I sowed will be watered by another, and soon be brought to harvest.

More than ever before, I recognize that every person we meet is somewhere on God's 24-hour clock. The first twelve hours is our life before knowing God's grace for us in Christ; conversion is that *kairos* moment that takes place at high noon; the second 12 hours is the time allotted as we are being sanctified. Grace based evangelism is being attentive to God's timing in a person's life. We then seek to help them to move the next fifteen minutes or half an hour, such that they receive more of the revelation of God's love for them in Christ.

My friend Kim, for instance, stopped with some of his buddies at a local Pizza Hut. When they got their order he said to his server, "God bless you." She rolled her eyes, and said, "Boys, I need that." Kim said, "Rough day?" She said, "You can say that again." "Rough day?"

He asked, "What's been so hard?" "You don't want to know." "I want to know." She looked at him again, wondering, one, if he was for real, and two, if it was worth the risk. She shared her heart; she was losing the war with a rebellious son. Kim is the youth pastor at the Toronto Airport Christian Fellowship, and after he had heard her out, he asked if he could pray for her. She asked, "Right here?" He checked out the floor behind her... and said, "Sure, here." "Father, let this dear lady know how much You love her. Let Your peace come upon her, and let her know that You love her son more than she does...."

When she opened her eyes, they were moist. She said, "That was wonderful! Thank you." He smiled, paid for his pizza, and left. Throughout the next day he prayed for her and on spec, returned with his friends to the same Pizza Hut the next evening... with a bouquet of roses. When he gave them to the waitress, she stared at it, stared at him, and then started to cry.

Kim did not have the privilege of speaking to her the noon-time word; he did play a significant role in moving her clock a half hour, even forty-five minutes closer, as she experienced care, prayer, and an open and generous heart, and equated it with a chance meeting with someone who named Jesus as his source.

Is this "compassion on the next one" something we have to work up? If it is, it will be "flesh giving birth to flesh."[7] One of the things we know in the midst of this outpouring is that what counts is what issues from the

[7] John 3.6.

overflow, rather than what gets dredged up from the bottom of our hearts. We have experienced deep within our hearts the love that God has lavished upon us; we have the deep conviction that He loves the person we are with more than we do; we have the confidence that the Spirit goes way before us, orchestrating and initiating encounters, such that there comes a meeting of heart to heart, even heart to Heart.

Again, it is ours to listen, two ways. We open our ears to the one we are with, recognizing that the unsaved are not one single and undifferentiated lump that needs to get converted. The Lord is at work in ways that are unique to each individual. It is for this reason that we open our hearts to what the Spirit is revealing and calling forth within us for the other. We ask, specifically, attentively, where a person is on God's clock, and how far the Lord purposes to take them. Having said that, we recognize that this is a time of boldness and favour. We are no longer just introducers. This is a season of accelerated grace.

Up and Out

En route to Japan, I was praying for my time there. My Bible reading had me in the latter chapters of Isaiah. Mid-Pacific, I lifted up God's promise of restoration from Isaiah 60.19-22: "The sun (I thought of Japan's flag) will no longer be your light by day... the Lord will be your everlasting light... and your days of mourning will be ended.... Your few will become a thousand; the handful, a great nation. At its appointed time I the Lord shall bring this swiftly to pass." With a deep stirring that this was an appointed time, I was both encouraged and expectant. "Lord, let your glory fall on this nation."

The last evening of the conference in Yokohama, I preached with a wonderful sense of boldness and authority, and when I gave the call for salvation, eleven put up their hands and came forward to receive Christ – something my missionary hosts said the Japanese did not do. What they did not understand quite yet is that in the midst of this outpouring of the Spirit, all the rules change!

What happened next surprised me, my team colleagues, our hosts, and the gathered congregation. We were in a large rented hall on the ninth floor of the Sogo department complex, reportedly the largest collection of stores in the world. That night, I had preached from 2 Kings 7, the story of the starving lepers who made their way into the deserted Aramean camp. After gorging themselves on the abandoned food and looting silver and gold, "they said to one another, 'What we are doing is not right. This is a day of good news, and we are keeping it to ourselves.'" I had spoken at length about the need to give away what we had received ourselves. By way of response, I asked those who knew that they had to share what they had received to stand. "Four desperate men were blessed beyond their wildest dreams, and knowing that what they had received, they had to share, they brought their people." I spoke of the text from Isaiah 60.22: "A few will become a thousand; the handful, a great nation. At its appointed time I the Lord shall bring this swiftly to pass." About a hundred and fifty men and women were soon on their feet. We prayed for them; we asked for evangelistic boldness, freedom, authority. We prayed that the Spirit would fill them and open doors that had long been shut. We prayed that the Lord would orchestrate divine appointments, and asked that the Spirit would be opening hearts to respond.

I then pointed to the doors of the hall. We sent these newly inducted evangelists out into the Sogo department stores, to tell good news. The rest of us stayed and interceded; we worshipped and had a ministry time. Within twenty minutes, many of the hundred and fifty had returned, several of them accompanied by brand new converts!

CHAPTER SIX

THE FIRE OF GOD'S LOVE:

Testimonies

... how immense are the resources of God's grace, and how great His kindness to us in Christ Jesus. Ephesians 2.7

* * *

The "Toronto Blessing" is but one of the ways God is currently pouring out His Spirit upon the Church. To name but a few of the other ministries that are also yielding notable evangelistic fruit, reports from Rodney Howard-Browne's "Revival Ministries International" cite 50,000 conversions from his international crusades in 1995. The Alpha course is an investigative group study aimed at those who want to know more about Christianity. It is home-based in Holy Trinity Brompton, London, and their office reports that there are four thousand courses now running worldwide, and that a quarter of a million people have worked through the course.

The Brownsville Assembly, in Pensacola Florida, marked 20,000 conversions on their first anniversary of protracted meetings, June 9th, 1995. And the men's movement, Promise Keepers, has called tens of thousands to commitment.

One of the songs that is frequently sung across these ministries is "The River of God," by Andy Park. The theme is taken from Ezekiel's vision in chapter 47: "I saw a spring of water issuing towards the east from under the threshold of the temple...." From what begins as a trickle, the river becomes an uncrossable torrent that flows out into the wastelands, reviving life, and bringing healing to the nations. A line in the song states that this river "brings refreshing, wherever it goes." We recognize that the river of the Father's grace is flowing in many, many different tributaries. The purpose of this chapter is to give an inside look to a few of the conversions that have resulted from the "Toronto Blessing."

* * *

Harley Esson, from a transcript of an interview conducted September, 1996.

Harley is thirty-four years old, and is presently a salesman for a photocopier company. He loves and honours his mum and dad, and recognizes that he grew up with parents who had been abused when they were children. His mother, particularly, was unable to bond emotionally with him.

Looking for love in all the wrong places, he married young; he was divorced two years later. He has a thirteen year old son from that marriage. Through his teen years and early twenties, he lived on the wild side. By way of drugs, he's used everything but needles. He frequently abused alcohol, in part to dull the emotional pain he carried. He has been repeatedly frustrated with his employment; his jobs never seemed to work out. Spiritually, he was raised as a nominal Catholic, and stopped going to church when he was nine. Until recently, Harley had a dim view of Christianity, and was wary of evangelicals and "born-againers." What put him off most was what he perceived as judgementalism.

Harley's pre-conversion boss was extremely wealthy. They spent a considerable amount of time together; part of Harley was enjoying the high living, high rolling lifestyle.

Another part was looking for something more.

As Harley testifies, he knows what it is to be lost; now, he knows what it is to be forgiven.

In mid-August of 1995, Harley was listening to his favourite talk show, AM 640, "Toronto Talks." The hosts, Horsman and Lederman, had visited "The Laughing Church," for it had recently been named the "Number one tourist attraction" in the magazine, *Toronto Life*. The show consisted of numerous interviews conducted with people who had *lined up* to get into the Toronto Airport Vineyard. That, in itself, caught Harley's attention. He'd never heard of a church that drew crowds like that. What really caught his attention was that he could hear joy in the voices of those interviewed. Sound clips from the worship were aired, and the music sounded great. There were interviews conducted inside, and Harley thought that all the talk about the "physical manifestations" sounded extremely strange. That was the conclusion the talk show hosts drew: "We don't understand what's going on here, but something is definitely happening." Harley agreed: "Wow, that would be something if it was true." In retrospect, Harley had thought once in a while about trying church again. He thought about the show on the Toronto Airport Vineyard for the next month. He wanted to go and see for himself, but felt he couldn't. He thought, "Jesus, if You're really there, I can't go until I clean up my life."

He talked to his mother about church, and remembers saying that the last thing he wanted to be was a "born-againer." Nevertheless, a couple of days later, he knew he "needed" to go to the Airport Vineyard. He knew his life wasn't headed in the right direction, and he was desperate for some measure of peace.

At his first meeting, he felt very nervous. Harley sat right at the back of the church, insurance in case he needed to make a quick exit. He positioned himself immediately in front of a structural support pillar, so that his backside was covered. Then he watched and waited: either, God was going to meet him, or, he'd quickly conclude that this deal was a fake. He was more than ready for a scam.

Harley watched as over a thousand people from all over the world sang their hearts out. He'd never seen people lift their hands while they worshipped. Part of him thought that they were showing off; another part could feel joy in the very air.

That night, pastor John Arnott preached on God's love, the love of a perfect Father. Harley had watched some TV religion; he'd heard the "turn or burn" messages. John's message was brand new.

At the conclusion of his sermon, John gave a short salvation message, and issued the call. Harley said to himself, "If that's true, then that's what I want." He didn't go forward in answer to John's invitation however. He didn't feel it was necessary. He was responding to what Harley called a "TV revulsion." He did, however, go to the back of the sanctuary, and take his place on one of the lines, waiting for prayer. Standing there, he was convinced that the falling down was all psychological. "God, I know that's not You, but I think You're here. I need You, and I need to know You're real. I need to know that everything they're telling me is real. Here I am."

Harley said that nothing happened. Nothing eventful, at least. He didn't fall down when someone on ministry team prayed for him. But driving home that night, he said he had the strangest feeling, like something was missing. When he parked his car in the driveway, it dawned on him: his anger was what was missing. It didn't make any sense. His driving habits had changed.

When he found himself in the slow lane, he wasn't cursing. He couldn't throw his cigarette butts out the window like he always had done previously. Out loud, he asked, "What's going on here??"

Harley went to the Toronto Airport Vineyard a second night, to try to make sense of the changes he felt were taking place. That, and the feeling that he knew he needed more. He knew that God was real. Moreover, Harley had a growing sense that God loved him; Harley wanted more of that love.

He especially watched people as they worshipped. Looking at a girl on her knees brought him to tears. The third night, he prayed, "God, it's so awesome that You're real. But Lord, if only I had a mother that could have held me." Shortly after that simple prayer, an elderly couple came in late, and sat down beside him. Towards the end of the worship, the woman leaned over, and spontaneously hugged Harley. As she held him in her arms, she told him that she loved him in Jesus. Harley was overwhelmed that God had heard and so quickly answered his prayer.

He kept going back. He was convinced that God was the source of the unusual manifestations. One night, Harley felt as if Jesus had asked him a question: "Why do you always come to My house depressed? Relax. I really like you. I've forgiven you; now, enjoy yourself." Later that night, Harley found himself asking, "Father, what do You want me to do?" By way of an answer, Harley heard the Lord speak to his heart: "I want you to quit smoking. It's hurting you." Harley made a deal: "OK. You help me with the nicotine addiction, and I'll quit." From that night on, Harley has had neither a cigarette, nor any alcohol.

One night, while resting on the floor after receiving prayer, he listened to a little girl who was laughing somewhere behind him. She was in hysterics for a half an hour. Harley suddenly realized that a little kid couldn't and wouldn't fake it for that long. Knowing then that this was for real, he asked for the holy laughter. But feeling unworthy, he believed the lie that only better, more mature Christians got it. Nevertheless, Harley kept coming, and coming, and coming.

He became so gloriously overwhelmed with the realization that "God is real!" and "Not only that, He does things!" that he lived in what he called "salvation shock" for several months. During this time, while nothing was happening by way of physical manifestations, God was transforming his life on a daily basis. For instance, while driving home alone in his car, the Holy Spirit revealed insights into his father's life, and why he couldn't extend to Harley the care he so longed for. "Your dad's father was a military man, and he showed no affection to your father as a child. You're just getting to know who your heavenly Father is, and your earthly dad doesn't yet know that love, so how can you expect your earthly father to give what he never received, and what your Heavenly Father can only give in fullness." In his head, Harley wondered, "Where did that come from?" What he clearly knows now is that this was the beginning of the process that enabled him to understand and forgive his father.

The more Harley went to the Toronto Airport Vineyard, the more desperate he became to feel God's love. He was trying so hard to receive. Someone on ministry team helped him be still, and quit striving. He worshipped quietly for several weeks, and then, one morning at the Burloak church plant, there were a number of prophetic words given during the worship. Harley found himself weeping. Later in the service, pastor Val Dodd said, "the Lord wants to give someone here a deep emotional healing today." Harley responded, going forward for prayer. The ministry team started praying in tongues over him, and he thought it was ridiculous. But he chose not to let it bother him. Minutes later, he found himself on his hands and knees. The person praying for him spoke out a prophetic word: "My son, I've called you out to join my priesthood." Harley's weeping turned into wailing. It felt like a vacuum cleaner was sucking out all the pain in his heart. And then, suddenly, his bawling turned into hysterics. Everyone else at the back of the hall, having coffee; alone, Harley enjoyed wave after wave of his Father's love, engulfing him. All he could do was laugh.

That same morning, Harley had given Barry, his father, a copy of John Arnott's video tape on the Father's love. Coincidentally, Barry's three appointments for the day were cancelled. Driving home, Harley prayed, "Please Lord, let my dad be home so that I can tell him what just happened this morning."

When Harley walked through the door, the video he had left with his father was just ending. Harley couldn't contain himself: "Dad, God's real!" The Holy Spirit fell on him again; this time, Harley was jerking with what seemed like electro-shock convulsions. He managed a stilted, "I'm okay, Dad; it's God." Watching his son, writhing on the kitchen floor, laughing, jerking, his father seriously considered calling the emergency services. He knew that Harley wasn't faking, and it freaked him a bit, to say the least.

Barry, came to one of the services at the Toronto Airport Vineyard a week or so later, to see what was going on. He was seemingly unaffected. He didn't go forward for prayer, and didn't say much about the meeting on the way home. All on his own a few nights later, Harley asked one of the ministry team, Doug, to join him in asking that the Holy Spirit would move on his father. Doug agreed to "agree" with Harley's prayers. "Holy Spirit, go get my dad, and bring him here. Free him from his pain and despair."

The next day, Harley got home from work, and before he could say anything, his dad said, "I'd like to go back to the Airport church with you." Driving there, Barry talked about how, for most of the day, he'd had this strange urge to go to the service that night. Once they pulled into the parking lot, Harley told his dad what he had prayed the night before.

Barry sat through the service, and again did not respond to the altar call. This time he did go to the back for prayer with his son. There, Harley prayed, "Please send Doug to us, because he knows what's going on here." He stood with his eyes closed for some time, and when he opened them, there was Doug, standing in front of them. "Doug, this is my dad!"

Doug told Barry how much Harley loved him. He started to pray for Barry, and Barry's flesh started to quiver. Doug asked Barry if he'd like to receive Jesus, and that night, Harley's dad gave his life to the Lord.

At a service a couple of weeks later, Barry went forward in response to the altar call, and made a public commitment to the Lord. Since then, his life evidences the power of God's grace upon it. He has been freed from his over-use of alcohol, and delivered from his depression and hopelessness. Barry is now a student of God's Word, and regularly attends one of the Toronto Airport Christian Fellowship's church plants, the Burloak Fellowship. He is part of one of their small groups, and has been to several of the Promise Keepers' local rallies. He is committed to seeing his family restored in Christ, and Harley can only say, "It's awesome."

In a conversation with his mother shortly after Harley started going to the church, Harley told her that he'd given his heart to Jesus. He then asked, "Mum, I want you to come to this church so that you know that it's not a cult, and that I haven't flipped out." She came that night, and said that she felt the Lord's presence there, but she didn't go forward for prayer. The next night, she went to a service at her Catholic church, a charismatic healing Mass, and when she got home at 1 o'clock in the morning, immediately called Harley. She had gone forward for prayer there, and when they had laid hands on her, she'd gotten completely inebriated in the Spirit. She said that right then and there, she knew that God loved *her*. A while later, the priest led her and the entire congregation through the sinner's prayer, and concluded by saying, "So, you're all born again now. What do you think of *that*?" Harley is amazed at the change that has come over his mother: she's on fire for the Lord; she frequently has spiritual dreams and visions, and is now actively involved at her Catholic church. Where Harley and his mum would go months without talking to each other, now they talk daily, mostly about the Lord. Harley is so grateful that what never bonded between them in the natural, the Lord is restoring in the Spirit.

About thirty days into his new life in Christ, Harley became friends with a pastoral couple from Michigan. They had come to the Airport church for a week, and while they were there, Harley spent considerable time with them. Before leaving, they invited him to come to a small town outside Flint to share his testimony with their congregation. A few weeks later Harley drove down and started telling the church about how awesome God is. "It could only be God who could take a guy who was raised Catholic but had never been in church since grade four, reveal Jesus to him, and then have him stand in front of a Baptist congregation a month later, telling them about the heart of the Father!"

Overcome with the Spirit's power and presence, he was soon on the floor, laughing, and feeling like electricity was jolting through him. Later, a lady came up to him and asked if he was going to be travelling in the future. "I get this strong feeling that the Lord's telling you not to." Harley didn't pay much attention. "Yeah, so...."

The next morning, he was back at work. His boss told him to go home, and pack a bag. "We're going to Pennsylvania in an hour," he explained. As he was packing, Harley remembered the Michigan lady's warning. Unheeding, he went back to work.

Ten years previously, Harley had been arrested for possession of narcotics. His criminal record had never been a problem at the border, because he'd never confessed it, and he'd never been the subject of a spot-check. This time, Harley knew it would be different, and why it was he shouldn't have been "travelling." He and his boss were called in by customs officials, and Harley was directly asked, "Do you have a criminal record?" Harley lied. His identity and history was checked on the computer. The customs official came back red-faced, yelling words like "fraud" and "fines" and "prison sentence." For the moment, they noted his infraction on the computer, and denied him entrance to the USA.

Harley said, "I was in a major repentance mode for weeks." A while later, the youth pastor from the church in Michigan called, to ask if Harley could come back in a month to speak to the teens. While knowing that he couldn't legally return, he had a strong sense of God's mercy and grace on his past life. So much so, that he said yes to the invitation.

A new US immigration law was passed in 1995, essentially granting amnesty for previous drug abusers. Besides $150, what was required was a complete disclosure of one's criminal record, current fingerprints, and medical declarations. There were letters to be secured from the Royal Canadian Mounted Police, and a letter from one's employer that clearly demonstrated that there were business imperatives that necessitated cross border travel. All of that was to be forwarded to the US Department of Justice, and, after a favourable hearing, a 60-day renewable entrance pass would be granted. Harley immediately began to gather the various documents that were required to make application for the amnesty, hoping that things would all be settled in time. He and his small group prayed fervently.

Harley was scheduled to leave on a Friday morning. At the Toronto Airport Vineyard on Thursday night, he again made full confession, and surrendered all of his hopes and plans: "Lord, if You don't want me to go, make my car break down. If this whole thing is a test of faith, make my car break down in Windsor, right before the border. If it's Your will that I go, blind the eyes of the customs officials."

When he got home after the meeting, one of the anticipated documents had arrived. It was the most important one, from the RCMP. Holding it in his hands, he asked, "Lord, did You really do what I think You've done?" He opened what was his criminal record, with his fingerprints appended. This is what he saw, in bold, capital letters, with quotation marks: **"NO RECORD."**

He fell to his knees, and said, "Lord, there really is nothing impossible for You. You really did clean my slate, and not just spiritually." His father was standing in front of him, and right then and there, the Spirit fell on both of them. They had their own little celebration – "Just think, the Creator of the Universe, and He pours out on you in your own living room!"

When he drove across the border the next day, no questions were asked. In Michigan, he met with the youth group, and while he was speaking, a blizzard hit. After the meeting, he was to follow his hosts home, but because it was snowing so hard, he mistakenly followed the wrong car. By the time he realized his mistake, he was miles out of town, and good and lost. At a gas station, he tried to get directions to the church, on the corners of Atherton and Gennesse. He was told, "They don't meet." The man at a local store didn't know where it was. Harley phoned his hosts, and as it was late, he said he'd book himself into a motel.

He couldn't find one that was open. Signs were now covered with snow, there was lots of black ice on the roads, and he was getting more and more frustrated. At last he found a motel that was open, and bunked down for the night.

The next morning, it was clear and sunny, a beautiful Sunday morning. On checking out, he realized he was right around the corner from the church. He heard in his heart the Lord say, "What a difference the light makes, eh?" He continued: "Last night was what life was like before I brought you in. You had an idea where you wanted to go, but didn't have a clue how to get there. You couldn't find your way by yourself, because you were in darkness. But when I brought you into the light, it was easy to read the signs, and know which way you're going."

Some time later, Harley was worshipping at home, alone, and felt the strong presence of the Spirit. He was laughing and crying, and heard Jesus saying that He was with him, and that He loved him. Then doubts started creeping into his mind. "This is the Creator of the Universe – here in my basement?" What then flashed into his mind was "Deuteronomy 4.7." As a young Christian, Harley had heard of Deuteronomy, but had never read it. In his new Bible, he found the passage: "What other nation is so great as to have their gods near them the way the Lord our God is near us whenever we pray to Him." And he knew that Jesus was telling him, "Yes, it really is Me right there, speaking to you, loving you." His doubts evaporated.

Harley's son lives with his mother, north of Toronto.

Joey goes to a Catholic school, and Harley wanted to bring him to the church. He was concerned what his ex-wife would think, and what Joey would feel about the manifestations. Harley prayed that if it wasn't the right timing, that the Lord would stop him from extending the invitation; his heart was to tell him all about Jesus. One weekend with his son, Harley said, "Joey, what if I told you that the Holy Spirit really was real, and that He does things, and He can touch you, and you can feel His presence." Joey said, "Well, if you believe in God, you kind of have to believe in the Holy Spirit don't you?" Harley cut to the chase, told him of his conversion, and then asked him if he wanted to go to the Airport Church with him that night.

The first night they were there, Harley had some parental anxieties about how distracted his thirteen-year-old seemed to be. Harley then felt the Lord say, "You've done your job; you've brought him here. Now leave him to Me; I'll take care of the rest." Later that night, Joey went forward to give his life to the Lord. When he got prayed for, he "rested" as many have done. Harley asked him what that felt like, expecting "Neat." What Joey answered was, "Safe." Now, six months later, Joey wants to go to the Airport Christian Fellowship any opportunity he gets, and often asks when they can go next. He often dances before the Lord during worship. Harley says that their relationship as father and son has deepened and become more intimate and loving. Joey's become more affectionate, and a few weeks ago, Joey told Harley that *he'd* changed for the better!

In June 1996, Harley was invited back to the church in Michigan as part of a Catch the Fire conference. Lynn Patch was part of the ministry team, and accompanied him en route. They pulled into a town called Port Huron for coffee, bypassing McDonald's and a Wendy's, turning left down a small side street, and stopped in front of a pretty dingy diner. Before they went in, Harley found himself praying grace, blessing, and angelic covering over the establishment. Harley went to the men's room, and on his return, overheard Lynn asking the girl behind the counter, "Do you know Jesus?" Immediately, the girl, Sally, started to tell them how she was struggling how to know Him, how to receive Him. They told her that she could do it right now, and she asked, "right here?" They suggested they go into the back of the store; Lynn took her back where they make the donuts, and Harley stayed out front, "minding the store." After Lynn led her in prayer, Sally started to cry. By the time the two of them came back out front, Sally was radiant. On the way back to the car, Harley recognized again, after the fact, how clearly he had heard from the Lord; just in the moment, he thought he was going to get a coffee.

As Harley has reflects on this encounter, he sees such a contrast to the times when he's tried to share his new love for the Lord with his friends and family at home. The contrast seems so marked. It is as though they haven't been prepared to receive his testimony; the Holy Spirit hasn't prepared their hearts, and they haven't sensed Him wooing them. Harley more than sees the difference when he responds to how the Spirit precedes him, and when, in his zeal, Harley's taken the lead.

Now, Harley asks that the Lord lead him to people that are prepared to hear what the Spirit calls forth. Two months ago, at his new job, Harley was sitting in a room with a partner, discussing the sales territories that had been assigned to them. His associate said, "Well, I'm just going to trust the Lord, and not worry about it." Harley asked, "You're a Christian?" His associate began to tell him that he frequents Muslim meetings, Hare Krishna meetings, Christian meetings.... Harley sensed an open door, and shared his testimony with him, finishing by saying, "The reason I think God gave me this job is so that I can tell the people I work with how much He loves them."

Harley then had to go out to his car to get a city map. On the back seat, he had a New Life tract, "How to be Born Again." He picked it up, and said, "Lord, I want to give this to my associate, but if it's not Your timing, I don't want to push him away. If it is Your timing, and You're reaching out to him, and You want him to have this pamphlet, I know You'll set it up." Harley put the tract in his back pocket.

On his return, he sat down, and within four minutes, his friend asked, "Harley, tell me something: what does

146

it mean to be born again?" "Way to go, God!" Harley mumbled under his breath, and leaned forward, pulled out the tract, and told the man exactly what he had prayed at his car, adding, "It's obvious that the Lord is reaching out to you, and He wants you to know that He loves you, and that His Son died for you. I really suggest that you open your heart to Him."

With that, he gave him the pamphlet. Their time together was then interrupted, and Harley left knowing that a Kingdom seed had been planted in some wonderfully prepared ground.

* * *

Harley gave some thought to all that's changed in his life. Here are his concluding reflections.

"My Father has just given me the revelation that regardless of what I am, and what I do, or don't do, He's totally enthralled with me. It makes no sense. That's where so many Christians have trouble. They try to make sense of it, and they can't ever understand it. All you can do is accept it. That revelation of how much your Heavenly Father really adores you, it's that that gives the release from the condemnation.

I know who I am if He were to lift His grace off my life. I know that His love is a free gift, and there is no possible way to cut a deal with Him. When the Holy Spirit brings the revelation of His grace to your heart, the most important thing is to receive it. The key to receiving it seems to be resisting the inclination to judge what we don't understand.

* * *

Stephan Witt, September 1996

At the time of this testimony, Steve was pastor of the Rothesay Vineyard outside Saint John, New Brunswick. He and his family had planted the work in 1986. Steve was experiencing the dryness of ministry in the winter of 1994; after a short sabbatical, he came to Toronto in April to investigate the reports circulating about the Toronto Airport Vineyard. God blessed him and his team mightily, as they were overcome by gutwrenching laughter and fresh vision for ministry. Steve's "seeker sensitive church," the Rothesay Vineyard, was radically shaken and soon became a renewal centre for the region, hosting multiple conferences. As many as 1,700 from many different denominations have attended. They have renewal services now in four Maritime cities where two church plants have been birthed. Renewal has energized teams that minister regularly.

In June of 1996, the Witt family felt called by the Lord to plant a church in Cleveland Ohio. The Metro Church South has emerged, and is working toward city renewal with other area pastors.[1]

* * *

[1] Metro Church South of Greater Cleveland (330) 225-9200; Email 105066.2505@Compuserve.com.

One day in late September 1995, I felt in desperate need of an undistracted prayer time. My home was off limits due to young children; the church office was too noisy because of our Christian school. I opted for a prayer walk. It wasn't as quiet as I thought it would be. Birds chirped, squirrels scurried about and everything seemed *busy*.

This particular walk took me to the parking lot of a local McDonald's, a teenage hangout in our community. On Fridays and Saturdays as many as 250 teenagers gather there and usually, there's trouble before the night's out. McDonald's management has repeatedly failed to find a workable solution.

As I approached, I noticed a group of teens arguing with a female manager of the restaurant. I walked up and inquired if I could help. She was clearly frustrated as she explained the futility of the situation. "There's nothing you can do," she shrugged. "There's nothing anyone can do." I introduced myself, and said, "I know a way to get the teens out of your parking lot." Doubt and cynicism looked me in the face as I continued. "We can bring a ministry team down here and tell the kids about Jesus!" A gleam of hope filled her eyes and with a raised finger she said, "*That* might work."

I hurried back to the church and shared the opportunity with my associate, Bruce Lindsay. Within twenty-four hours we had a team ready for our first "McMission." At our regular Friday night renewal service, we explained the situation to the congregation, and seven men volunteered to serve. We prayed for them and sent them out.

Our church had been experiencing "Toronto Blessing" renewal for six months. We had witnessed the falling on the floor, the hysterical laughter, the shaking, weeping, angelic sightings and more. It was now time to discover if this was something more than just experience; had lives been changed, and had something been imparted? That Friday night's renewal meeting was our launch pad for some bold "confrontational evangelism." Boldness was unquestionably one of the characteristics of the early Church after Pentecost.[2] Some of those we sent out had never faced hard core, toe to toe evangelism like this, where *we* took the initiative.

One hundred and fifty people interceded as the McMission team went out. While we were worshipping, our renewal service was interrupted as seven teens stormed into the church lobby. They were running from a gang of kids armed with baseball bats. Just fifteen minutes earlier, we had prayed that the youth of our city would be attracted to our church and find it a refuge, but we never expected such an immediate answer! Someone commented, "We've sown a team to McDonald's and reaped an outreach in our own backyard!"

A little later, the police came by the church to deal

---

[2] See Acts 2.14; 4.8-13; 4.31; 9.17-29; 13.9-10, 46; 18.26; 19.8; 28.31

with the problem teenagers with the baseball bats. As the officer stepped out of his car, he looked at me and said, "You have no idea the impact you had on those teens at McDonald's." As it happened, this particular officer had observed the McMission, and was the first to bring a favourable report.

Just then the team returned from McDonald's and as we went inside, we swapped stories. When our team had arrived at McDonald's, they quietly filtered into the crowd, asking questions, trying to establish relationship with the teens. There was no sound system for any worship, nor tracts to be handed out, just "renewed" men full of Holy Spirit boldness, drawing on the deposit of hours of carpet time.

One of the team members offered to pray for one of the kids. The teenager began to shake. That was a common phenomenon in our church, but not in a McDonald's parking lot. This was a very different kind of Big Mac attack! As he kept shaking, those looking on responded, "Cool!" "Do it to me, do it to me!!!"

Prayer, counsel and encouragement ensued for hours, as our men helped a number of the teens with general issues of life. One young man gave his life to the Lord, and others were genuinely touched by the love of the "McMissionaries."

We had several other McMissions while the weather allowed it. One week, we distributed free hot dogs in an adjacent parking lot, just to show God's love in a practical way. This ministry was only for a season;

we're no longer doing McMissions, because the problem with teens gathering has been resolved. Looking back on our time there, we feel that there were two key fruits harvested. First, our people were given an opportunity to let the renewal river flow out from the church and into the streets. We have a keener awareness of the needs in our city, and an expectant sense that the Lord will continue to show us creative ways to touch them. Outreach is becoming as normal to our church as breathing is to any human. As part of two recent conferences, we went out into some of the poorer sections of our city. On one outreach, some of our people went door to door distributing light bulbs to the needy. One home that was visited had only one working bulb in the entire house! There, our team was invited in after they shared the purpose of the call. In the moments that followed they were given the privilege of praying for a single mother and her young child. With tears, she received the free box of light bulbs *and* the light of God. Our team was so overwhelmed, they gave her every light bulb they had!

They returned to this lady's house a while later; she'd asked for some information about our church. The team was deeply moved when they saw her home, once dark, now lit up with the light bulbs she'd received. What meant even more to them was that they knew it was the same in her heart!

The second result we've seen from McMission is that our immediate community was made aware of who we are, and what we stand for. There is a far greater sense of our "presence," and that our doors are open to those who are looking for a safe place, a place that cares, a place where God is real. We believe that this, in part, was why we were able to draw sixty-five new believers and non-Christians to a recent Alpha Course that was based from our church.

We didn't see a great flood of souls from the McMission, but we celebrated a great flood of joy as the Word went forth. We leave the unknown results to the Lord.

* * *

The renewal has acted as a fuel for the vehicle of our local church. Whatever God used us in before is now "supercharged" as a result of soaking in His presence. Intercessors pray with fresh power, evangelists share with greater boldness, and pastors lead with greater liberty!

The Lord tailor-made McMission for us, for a short season. In the midst of this outpouring of the Spirit, each local church must "hear what the Spirit is saying to the church,"[3] and walk *that* out. This is not a time for "rubber stamping" of methods and copying what's worked somewhere else. Rather, we encourage one another with our stories of how the Spirit is working

---

[3] Revelation 2.29.

ahead of us. We attend to what is being called forth in our midst, and we customize a Spirit-led plan for our local situation. McMission was a flexible, simple response such that God's river of blessing could flow... out into the streets where it is the driest! Over those few Friday nights in the McDonald's parking lot, we touched the hearts of some teens; the larger consequence is that we as a local church saw that the "river" flows out from the "throne," into the streets, to bring healing. If we can see Christians around the world awakened to show God's love in practical ways... who knows, maybe "billions will be served!"

* * *

Steve Phillips, September 1996
Until recently, Steve was a Vineyard Area Overseer for fourteen churches in the US Midwest. This included Randy Clark's church in St. Louis, Missouri. Because of his overseer role with Randy, he was involved in the current renewal from the very start. He served at the Toronto meetings a few days after the renewal began in January 1994, and has preached there numerous times since. He now travels and teaches full-time with Equipping Ministries International, a prophetic/ evangelistic equipping ministry based out of the St. Louis Vineyard.

In March 1996, I was part of the leadership team for

the "Catch the Fire – Moscow" meetings which brought over 850 Russian pastors and their spouses together for three days of mighty outpourings.

One afternoon, during a workshop at the conference, I heard one of the speakers say, "Jesus once spat in someone's eye and it was healed." The preacher's point was that God sometimes asks us to do "unusual" things for Him. A moment later, I felt the Holy Spirit ask me if I would be willing to spit in someone's eye! Suddenly, all of the religious veneer of that Biblical scene was stripped away as I began to think about what it would be like to actually do such a thing. I thought at length about what I would feel like if I spit in someone's eye and they were not healed. How embarrassing and humiliating that would be!

I then began to weep as I thought that obedience to God sometimes requires humility to the point of humiliation. Through the tears and with faith only the size of a mustard seed, I said, "Yes, God, if You ask me to do that I would be willing to, even if I felt potentially humiliated. But please – let me hear Your voice clearly!"

Fifteen minutes later, I was asked to minister on stage and, as you might guess, our hosts brought me a young girl in her twenties who had been in a coma earlier that year. We were told that she had been on the verge of death. Through the prayers of her church, God had miraculously raised her up. The only remaining legacy of her ordeal was blindness in one eye. Immediately I felt the Lord say, "This is the one!" My heart sank. "Oh, God, does it have to be a woman? If I have to spit in someone's eye, couldn't it at least be some rugged old man? Besides, Father, she can see everything I'm about to do out of her good eye! I thought You meant they would be completely blind or at least they wouldn't be able to see me actually spit on them!"

All I felt in reply to my whining was Jesus' love for this precious young girl and His gentle prompting to proceed. I asked her if she would allow me to do whatever I felt God was saying to do. "Of course," she told the interpreter. As my tears began to flow again, I asked her to please close her good eye. (I simply could not bear to have the woman watch me spit in her face.) She looked more like an angel than a human as she stood there in simple faith, with only her blind eye open.

At that moment, I began to think, "Just how do you go about this sort of thing?" As I pursed my lips, ready to literally spit across open air space, I felt the Lord suggest, "You can spit on your fingers, if you like, and wipe it into her eye." Grateful for this partial reprieve, I proceeded to spit on my fingers and wipe it into her open eye!

The woman who had brought the blind woman to the stage began to weep. She then fell to the floor. She was immediately followed by the interpreter. Shortly thereafter, I followed. The young woman stood motionless for a few minutes waiting before God, until she too fell to the floor. We lay there sprawled out on the floor in front of the crowd for several minutes. To me, it seemed more like several years. Eventually the young woman sat up and closed her good eye. I heard her speak one word in Russian, and then heard the interpreter gasp. "She just said, 'Light!' She can see light!"

We were suddenly inundated by a rush of people from the audience who needed healing – many of them came forward with severe eye problems. As we prayed for the next couple hours, numerous people reported either complete or partial healing, including one elderly lady with cataracts so bad that she was unable to read her Bible two inches in front of her face. After prayer, she was reading sheet music that we held up over six feet away. Pandemonium broke out as we watched faith increasing in hundreds of people. We stood rejoicing in the goodness of our God.

We left Moscow to travel to other cities in outer Russia, and as we ministered, we shared this testimony. In Rostov-na-Donu, near the Black Sea, a former philosophy professor from Moscow University was healed after hearing this story. When she shared her testimony, over sixty people accepted the Lord. We left the next day with a new church planted in only three days!

I don't know what would have happened if I had been unwilling to do something as objectionable as spitting in a young girl's eye. I do know that I am so grateful that I did not miss seeing the Father heal these precious people. I sincerely hope that this testimony does not create a rash of weird behaviour devoid of sincerity, humility and maturity. The last thing we need is for everyone to start spitting in people's eyes! But I do trust that sharing this experience will encourage others to listen carefully to the leadings of the Lord with the simplicity that is willing to suffer potential humiliation for the sake of Christ, in order that more of Christ's Kingdom may be manifested in our midst, and in our day.

* * *

Norma and Richard Iredale, Edinburgh, Scotland, October 1996

Norma teaches English and Social Education in a Secondary School in a small town outside Edinburgh. She also runs the Scripture Union which provides Christian teaching for pupils on a voluntary basis. Norma's work in the school has been recognized and respected by local Christians from several churches who have prayed for the work for a number of years. Richard has been in full-time ministry for the past six years. His special emphasis has been on renewal, evangelism, and corporate prayer for revival. He is currently on the leadership team of a new Pentecostal church in Edinburgh.

Richard and Norma met each other through renewal, and were married in May, 1996.

In October 1994 Jim Paul brought a ministry team from the Toronto Airport Vineyard to Edinburgh and held a week of meetings. By the third day Norma was so overcome by the power of the Spirit that she spent most of the meeting on the floor. She also started to "jerk" a phenomenon common with those overwhelmed by God's presence. She began to wonder what would happen if the manifestations were to occur outside the church setting. She was soon to find out!

On the Friday morning of that week, Norma was studying Act 3 of Romeo and Juliet with her 6th year class. As she walked over to one boy to check his work, she began shaking and jerking violently and had to sit down. The pupils thought she was having a fit! Norma assured them that everything was okay and that this was "simply" the Spirit of God touching her. That got their attention and Norma was able to explain that God was near to them and wanted to be real in their lives. She got up and walked towards another boy who happened to be the only Christian that she knew of in the class. Once again she began to shake and was unable to get near him. She thought it must be amusing for those watching, as it appeared as if the boy had some sort of "force field" around him that she could not penetrate.

At this point God showed her something about the first boy. She asked him if he had once made a commitment to Christ when he was younger but had since turned away. The boy confirmed that this was the case. She was able to take this opportunity to explain something of the Gospel and the love of God, and then answer several of the students' questions. One of the girls walked out saying it was too "freaky" for her, but by the next week she started attending the lunch-time Scripture Union meetings with a friend she had brought along. She later gave her life to Christ. Of the fifteen pupils in the class, seven subsequently came to Christian meetings and six gave their lives to the Lord.

Soon after this incident other students began asking questions about God. During one Social Education class, one particular girl took the lead. Her first question was about teachers' maternity leave; the fourth was, "How can I be sure I am not going to hell?" Since the question was asked in that context, Norma felt free to answer her in front of the whole class and explained that salvation comes through faith in Christ. Several pupils remained behind to ask more questions, and one asked to be taken to church. That pupil came and gave her life to Jesus. The following week she brought a friend who did the same.

At the end of April 1995, Norma invited Richard Iredale, one of the Elders of the church she was attending, to come to the school to speak. During a ministry time, Richard invited the Holy Spirit to come as he prayed for several youngsters, most of whom ended up on the floor under the power of God. This seemed to usher in an even more powerful move of the Spirit in the school. Richard and Norma began a series of "Times of Refreshing" meetings after school which carried on into the summer holidays. The numbers coming to the lunch-time Scripture Union meetings rose from about a dozen to over twenty as pupils developed a keener interest in knowing more about God.

Richard picks up the story.

Over a period of about three months, sixteen young people made commitments to Christ. Others who were already Christians were renewed in their faith and developed a greater desire to follow the Lord. The "Times of Refreshing" meetings were never large but God always poured out His Spirit when we met. It became a familiar pattern: unsaved youngsters or "lukewarm" young Christians would come into the meeting to see what was going on. We would begin with worship, move into a time of teaching from the Bible, and then open up for prayer. God's Spirit would impact the lives of those who were there, particularly the unsaved! Many would end up on the floor under the power of God, knowing that He was real. Subsequently, they would give their lives to Christ.

I wish we could say that it was all plain sailing from then on, but that was not the case. A measure of persecution rose up against the work. This was led by local Christians opposed to the "Toronto Blessing." We were repeatedly accused of being a cult and although two of the local ministers supported us, the young people and Norma came under increasing pressure. At times this was particularly vehement. Norma was "investigated" by Scripture Union, the national body under whose auspices she had held the voluntary lunch time meetings for sixteen years. Although she and her associate Anne were totally exonerated and the "Times of Refreshing" meetings were separate and not under the auspices of Scripture Union, it was felt that the meetings should continue outside the school to prevent any embarrassment to the school officials. The pressure on the young people became great, both from parents and peers. Several stopped coming as a result.

The next weeks held more disappointment. Despite starting a discipleship group in a home, some of the youth began to drop away because of the increasing peer and parental pressure. For some, it seemed that commitment simply waned. We were left with a much smaller group of eight or nine whose commitment was such that they would follow the Lord, and were prepared to ride out the criticism.

In the spring of 1996 we started a monthly outreach at the local youth community centre known as the "Hutz." The young Christians played a major part in this. The outreach consisted of a band playing contemporary Christian music, drama, testimonies and a short evangelistic message. A group of five young teenage girls came to the second of these. They liked the music and were interested in the dramas, testimonies and message, but there was no response to the appeal for salvation. We decided to pray for some people. As we invited the Holy Spirit to come, a few Christians began to manifest the holy laughter and the "jerks." Everyone we prayed for ended up on the floor under the power of God. This immediately grabbed the attention of the unsaved teenagers. They decided they wanted to be prayed for too, but not in public. We took them into a smaller room, and explained something of the Gospel and God's love for them. We then prayed for them. They were all powerfully impacted by the Spirit of God and lay prostrate for some time under His power. Following this, four of the girls went home and asked Jesus into their lives and at the next after school meeting brought along another friend, who subsequently asked the Lord into her heart. Again, a very strong persecution rose against these new Christians, and one was immediately prevented from coming to further meetings. Of the five who made commitments, three are currently going on with God, coming to church and to the discipleship group.

It was interesting to us that once again it was the dynamic power and intervention of the Holy Spirit that "caught" these young "fish." Although the initial draw was the music, drama, testimonies and message, it was when the power of God was manifested that they were really caught. Though the numbers coming to Christ and remaining in Him have not been large, they are still more than we have ever seen before. The young disciples group continues and it is a great blessing to see their commitment to Christ. In July 1996, we took them on mission to Dublin in Southern Ireland. It was wonderful to see God use them as they shared the Gospel and prayed for people and saw some give their lives to Christ.

* * *

Michael Thompson, April 1995

Michael is presently the senior pastor of the Tabernacle, a non-denominational, charismatic fellowship on the Space Coast of Florida. He served for ten years as a denominational pastor before joining Jamie Buckingham's staff at the Tab. He was profoundly touched at the first Catch The Fire Conference in Toronto and joined a trans-denominational leadership team which brought Randy Clark to Melbourne.

Renewal dropped like a bomb in Brevard County, a small finger of land along the Atlantic coast in Central Florida, in January 1995. A year earlier, a small group of pastors had crossed denominational and racial lines to form a prayer coalition to cry out for revival in the county. Relationships of trust and credibility had been forming across all kinds of distinct theological and methodological lines to create a fertile seedbed for a sweeping move of God.

In October 1994, during the first "Catch The Fire" conference hosted in Toronto, four hungry but sceptical pastors from Melbourne ventured out to check out what God was reportedly doing in "the Blessing." Each of us received so much more than we anticipated, and, upon our return, the fire fell on each of our respective churches. Planning began immediately: meetings in the new year were scheduled with Randy Clark, from St. Louis. Expectations began to grow during Advent 1994 – the sense was that January would be explosive. January 1, 1995 surprised even the most optimistic! When the fire hit Melbourne, it landed on some dry tinder – pastors – who were desperate for the reality of the Kingdom and its commensurate signs of life.

A powerful expression of united renewal began that first evening, and continues today. For the first ten months services were held six nights a week at the Tabernacle auditorium. They were sponsored jointly by over a dozen Brevard County churches – Charismatic, Southern Baptist, United Methodist, and Presbyterian – a partial list of the denominational spectrum represented. Pastors and worship teams from many churches operated under the leadership of local Vineyard Pastor, Fred Grewe and a team of pastors who had been given the challenging responsibility of trying to "steward" the renewal. Services continue to be held on Friday evenings, with monthly protracted meetings to fan the flame. Renewal leaders from around the world have been to Melbourne, both to contribute to fuel the fires of renewal, and to see the model of pastoral unity God has forged.

Early on in the renewal meetings it became evident that this group of people – literally thousands who passed through the Tabernacle on a regular basis – were not content with an experiential joy-fest without the accompanying signs of the Kingdom. Jesus' mission to "preach the Gospel to the poor" became a heart-cry of the renewal leadership, and was quickly caught and readily embraced by the renewed saints in Brevard.

The first response was called forth when a local AIDS ministry, "Light of the Lord," and a ministry to the homeless, "Resurrection Ranch," came into financial crisis. One of the local pastors suggested that one of the renewal offerings should be given to these ministries. Even though the renewal itself was just getting established and still trying to get its fiscal feet on the ground, the decision was both unanimous and enthusiastic. The congregation was told of the need, and the offering received in that evening service was the largest single offering of the first quarter in renewal – $3,300 was given to help the homeless and hurting in the county.

That event served only to whet the appetite of the Melbourne Renewal's leadership, for what could be done together. It soon became apparent that the combined effort of renewed and united churches could equal far more than the sum of their individual parts. What individual bodies struggled and so often failed to do alone, the community of revived believers could successfully do together. Touching something of the unity that Jesus prayed for in John 17, we found ourselves the heirs of "commanded blessing" spoken of in Psalm 133.3. The Renewal leadership quickly realized this dynamic principle of spiritual growth and maturity for the larger Body of Christ, as they continued to gather and work together.

The ministry to the poor emerging from Melbourne represents some of the "fruit" of renewed lives. It has risen "naturally-supernaturally" from the hearts of those who have opened their hearts, and received this fresh outpouring of God's Spirit. From the early days of the renewal, there has been a desire for a river of God to flow consistently and lovingly from the house of the Lord, out to the desert places. Such was the case when God began to speak to the leaders again during their first "Catch The Fire" conference, in August 1995.

The conference drew leaders such as Southern Baptist leaders, Peter Lord and Jack Taylor, from Florida; Guy Chevreau, from Toronto; David Ruis, from Winnipeg; everyone was delighted at Randy Clark's return. Scheduled as a conference, registrations covered costs, and no offerings were planned. But in the middle of the week, the Lord stirred the leaders to ask the congregation for an offering for various ministries to the poor in Brevard county. Over $10,000 was given in the single offering, received the second last night of the conference. From that offering, the homeless and AIDS ministries were again blessed, and an outreach to feed street people was funded. God also gave birth to "Project Light," an on-going ministry to kids, in the government housing projects.

Roger Hackenburg and Marc Telesha, Pastors of the Lighthouse Assembly of God, worked with a group of people from 10 local Melbourne churches, and began an outreach in one of the nearby housing projects. In a ministry that combines social action and Gospel preaching, volunteers stepped out of their comfort zones, and into the battle zones of the county. A children's music, puppet and game program is combined with a relevant and fast-paced presentation of the Gospel. While this ministry is aimed at the children, food, clothes and practical social aid is made available for families at each event.

As credibility is built by consistency, sceptical adults have joined the children who come. Both children and adults have accepted Christ; the Gospel has been incarnated among the poor. The unity of the churches and their lack of competition is amazing to those who watch. They've never seen the reality of Christ's united Body so clearly and generously demonstrated.

The ministry began in one section of town known for its violence and drug traffic. Not only has it been received, but even the police have gotten in on the act! Sidewalk Sunday School has grown to two locations – one in conjunction with a local church in the neighbourhood. Crossing racial and cultural lines, the love shared has been contagious. Invitations stand at present for at least three more locations.

Over $6,000 from Renewal funds have been invested in this ministry, purchasing sound equipment, outfitting a trailer and providing food to be given away. Most of the more than sixty regular volunteers have risen from the ranks of the "carpet time" brigade. This united effort has arisen like a phoenix from the fires of renewal! With the passion generated by these outreaches, Hackenburg and crew sponsored an Operation Blessing outreach. Taking many middle-class suburbanites out of their familiar surroundings, the loving workers invaded one of Melbourne's toughest neighbourhoods. Gospel music blared over loudspeakers as nearly four hundred workers from thirty-six churches gave out 40,000 pounds of food to nearly 3,000 families. Because of the atmosphere of love and unity, one hundred and forty people were bold enough to receive prayer and forty of them accepted Christ for the first time in their lives.

The saga continues! On Yom Kippur 1995, the Melbourne Renewal invited other Evangelicals to join them for a prayer meeting at the Space Coast Stadium. Over 3,500 brave souls defied pouring rain to gather and pray for revival in the county. An offering was received and all of it went to the ministries to the poor in the county. The Renewal covered over $3,500 in expenses so that the joint offering, nearly $14,000, could be given away. Two local Habitat for Humanity chapters were supported. (This is a co-operative organization that builds low cost housing.) A food kitchen, food bank and community development agency were also blessed with financial aid.

Out of relationships built in renewal, meetings were sponsored by a small, African-American congregation in the heart of the drug district. Area pastors took turns preaching, leading worship, and praying in services that dwarfed the expectations of all who were involved in their planning. Unity across denominational and racial lines has lead to co-operation in both evangelistic and social action efforts in the community. Not only is the fire catching, but so is the vision for what happens when renewed people take their fresh life to the strongholds in society.

It has become increasingly clear in the Melbourne Renewal that if the powerful exhibition of the life of God doesn't give an even more powerful expression of the heart of God, it is a myopic move which will be short-lived. God is not merely into entertaining the troops. His desire is that the dry bones rise up as an exceeding great army to do battle for the hearts of men and the soul of the nations.

We've seen significant demonstrations of this locally. One of the Melbourne area churches affected deeply by renewal had made many concrete attempts to cross boundaries and break barriers to demonstrate the reality of the love and unity of Christ. A middle-aged white Southern Baptist pastor hired a fiery black Pentecostal as his associate pastor. The church longed for their associate to be full-time, but the money wasn't yet there to fully support him. One day in the Renewal Pastor's meeting the Pastor came in to share that his associate had run into a major financial need. Before he left the meeting that day, $800 was placed in his hands by caring leaders. Shortly thereafter, the Renewal leadership approved an $800 per month stipend for six months to help this brother get established. The ministry of reconciliation was pragmatically underway.

The Melbourne renewal churches were also privileged to play a part in a Russian outreach. After a challenge by Randy Clark, we raised over $5,000 to sponsor Russian church leaders as they gathered for a renewal conference in Moscow. On top of that, over $6,000 came in to support pastors who were planting churches out of renewal throughout the former Soviet Union.

Renewal has made an impact to the south of us as well. On a routine trip to Honduras to ferret out potential development project sights, our missionary pastor, Jonathan Smoak, discovered that during seasons of renewal nothing is routine!

Community development and relief was a part of the growing missions strategy of the Tabernacle Church in Melbourne before renewal fires blazed hot in the county. After prophetic promptings from leadership, the search team for a 1995 summer Honduras project went away thinking that perhaps something was up.

Upon arrival in Honduras, and giving in to gentle promptings of the Spirit, the team went to evaluate a Christian camp – Bethel – as the possible destination spot for a Junior High discipleship trip. Smoak had led development projects in Honduras dozens of times, but had never been to this particular camp. He knocked on the door of the home which housed Bethel's overseers. A stately lady named Elva greeted them, and began to discuss the business of the camp – in Spanish.

When the project was proposed, there was hesitance on Elva's part; she was protective of the beautiful facility – an enigma in the drab and poverty-stricken Honduran culture. But another gentle prompting from the Spirit caused Jonathan to ask her if she'd ever heard of Jamie Buckingham, a prolific Charismatic writer and the Tabernacle's founding pastor. Immediately, Elva began to speak flawless English and reported how indebted she'd been to Jamie's writings.

The door was swung wide open for the missions/ discipleship trip! As the discussion continued, Elva suggested that the team look at the facilities – which were more than adequate for the needs of the planned trip. When they walked into the auditorium, the team nearly fainted. The building was an absolute duplicate of the Tabernacle's Melbourne auditorium. Smoak breathlessly reported to Elva, "This is our church!" She replied, "Yes. I was at the Tabernacle nearly a dozen years ago and fell in love with the simplicity and size of the building. We were in the development stages of Camp Bethel, so we duplicated the building we'd seen."

It was then that the divine pieces began to come together. Elva reported that the camp had been built with the vision of being a renewal centre for leaders in

Honduras. She stated that for nearly a dozen years she had waited and prayed, watching as the camp was used for many good things, but never for leadership revival. She had heard reports of renewal in Toronto, but their limited resources made it impossible for them to travel that far. She had heard reports from nearby Melbourne, and had been praying for someone to come from there and share the fire! Now, Jonathan was standing on her doorstep – renewal was just around the corner.

From those sovereignly orchestrated beginnings, the Melbourne Renewal Fellowship began to pursue ongoing relationships with leaders in the Honduran church. At the end of May, 1995, the Renewal underwrote the costs to bring twenty-five Honduran leaders to a week of meetings in Melbourne. Subsequently, in October, a "Catch The Fire" conference featuring trans-denominational leaders from Melbourne was held at Bethel; a second conference was hosted in the summer of 1996.

Twelve years ago, at Bethel's inception, revival seeds were planted. What an awesome privilege it has been to see God harvest fruit as events in Toronto, Melbourne and Honduras catalyzed, such that one hundred and fifty Honduran leaders came into such a powerful ministry of the Holy Spirit, and equally dynamic youth renewal meetings brought great joy to young people from churches across Tegucigalpa during the Junior High trip, the original reason for finding Bethel.

* * *

Since the beginnings of renewal in Melbourne, God seems to have directed much of the spiritual energy and refreshment to ministry to the poor, to the marginalized in the county, and on overseas mission fields in Honduras and Russia. Whether in the neighbourhood, in the struggling church or in a foreign land, renewal in Melbourne has resulted in a passion for the Kingdom and its expression to the poor. The stories are so easy to multiply. Recently, six beach-side churches joined together to build a Habitat for Humanity house for a needy family in the area. The Baptist pastor leading the push stated emphatically, "This happened as direct fruit of the Renewal." A medical and teaching team is preparing for the second "Catch The Fire" conference in Honduras for 1996.

In so many ways, Melbourne Renewal seems to be a reflection of the first miracle that Jesus performed. In John 2, at the wedding feast in Cana, the party had run dry. This fact was lamented, and in response, Jesus commanded that the ceremonial pots be filled with water; when it was poured out, the water had become the finest of wine!

Jesus heard the desperate cries of pastors and people in Melbourne for a move of His Spirit. He reached across denominational lines and filled whatever ceremonial vessels (traditions, creeds, worship styles) that were empty and desperate enough to receive. We have been filled to overflowing with the water of life. As He has poured us out, we have become an intoxicating and aromatic fragrance, a revelation of the heart and compassion of Christ, especially to the hurting!

* * *

Nearly five hundred years ago, reformation swept the Church in Europe. We are seeing a wonderful reformation of faith and witness in our day. Ours is such a rich heritage. Martin Luther, in his famous *Preface to Romans*, gave us language to speak of all that is ours in Christ:

> Faith is a living, daring confidence in God's grace, so sure and certain that the believer would stake his life on it a thousand times. This knowledge of and confidence in God's grace makes men glad and bold and happy in dealing with God and with all creatures. And this is the work which the Holy Spirit performs in faith. Because of it, without compulsion, a person is ready and glad to do good to everyone, to serve everyone, to suffer everything, out of love and praise to God who has shown him this grace.[4]

[4] Luther's Works, vol.35, *Word and Sacrament*, Concordia Pub. House, St. Louis, 1963, p.371.

SOAKING WITH PURPOSE

I will venture to speak only of what Christ has done through me to bring the Gentiles into His allegiance, by word and deed, by the power of signs and wonders, and by the power of the Holy Spirit. Romans 15.18-19

* * *

Ninety years ago, the meetings at 312 Azusa Street commanded considerable press coverage. Unlike the media favour that has characterized the reports of the "Toronto Blessing," this secular newspaper article is representative of the prejudices brought against the first Pentecostals:

> There is a most disgraceful intermingling of the races. Together, they cry and make howling noises all day and into the night. They run, jump, shake all over, shout to the top of their voice, spin around in circles, fall out on the sawdust blanketed floor jerking, kicking and rolling all over it. Some of them pass out and do not move for hours as though they were dead. These people appear to be mad,

176

mentally deranged or under a spell. They claim to be filled with the Spirit.

They have a one-eyed, illiterate Negro as their preacher who stays on his knees much of the time with his head hidden between wooden milk crates [his pulpit]. He doesn't talk very much but at times he can be heard shouting "Repent," and he's supposed to be running the thing.... They repeatedly sing the same song, 'The Comforter Has Come.' [1]

Pastor Frank Bartleman chronicled the birth of Pentecostalism. He described some of the dynamics of the meetings held in the "tumble-down shack" on Azusa Street:

The services ran almost continuously. Seeking souls could be found under the power almost any hour, night and day. The place was never closed nor empty. The people came to meet God. He was always there. Hence a continuous meeting. The meeting did not depend on the human leader. God's presence became more and more wonderful. In that old building, with its low rafters and bare floors, God took strong men and women to pieces, and put them together again, for His glory. It

[1] Art Glass, *Pentecostal Heritage, Inc.*, unpublished paper, Pentecostal Azusa Revival Museum, p.8.

was a tremendous overhauling process. Pride and self-assertion, self-importance and self-esteem, could not survive there.[2]

It is estimated that thirteen thousand leaders came to the meetings on Azusa Street. Those whom God "took to pieces" returned to their respective homes, and nearly a hundred years later, the fruit of their lives and ministries represents the greatest evangelistic and missionary enterprise Christendom has ever witnessed – it is estimated that there are now half a billion Pentecostals/Charismatics worldwide.

In the midst of this present outpouring of God's Spirit, thousands would concur with Bartleman's observations: God has overhauled us; first, we have been taken to pieces, and then put together again for His glory. Pride, performance, insecurity, fear, competitiveness and issues of control are being healed and redeemed. This work is so deep, and so profound that many of us struggle to give expression to the grace we have touched, and the life-transformations that have been called forth.

The Last of the Fathers

Chapter One of *Share The Fire* closed with a quotation by Bernard of Clairvaux. Bernard is an

[2] Frank Bartleman, *How Pentecost Came to Los Angeles: As It Was In The Beginning*, 2nd Ed. (Los Angeles: By the Author, 1925), p.58.

important figure in the history of the Church for many reasons; among them that he was able to give expression to the most intimate of revelations received from the Lord. He was so articulate that he earned the title: "Mellifluous Doctor," "the Doctor-flowing-with-honey."

For Bernard, theology rose out of meditation and prayer, loving devotion and revelation. Heir of the rich monastic tradition of John Cassian and Benedict, Bernard's understanding and experience of God's love was grounded in worship, and characterized by the maxim: *Semper in ore psalmus, semper in corde Christus,* "Always a psalm on the lips, always Christ in the heart."

Bernard was not just a writer of spiritual theology though; he had tremendous influence on the political, literary and religious life of Europe, and is known as one of the great revivalists and reformers of the High Middle Ages. It is said of Bernard that "he cast fire on earth wherever he went. God worked in him, and worked such wonders that men knew it was God they had seen at work, not man. The grace of the God who had possession of this frail man burst into flame in the hearts of all who heard him speak."[3]

In 1113, at the age of 22, Bernard entered a floundering new monastery at Citeaux. His influence

---

[3] Thomas Merton, *The Last of the Fathers.* Harcourt Brace Jovanovich, Pub., New York, 1954, p.27.

was such that he brought thirty friends and relatives with him, more than doubling the community's size. Four years later, he was elected to lead a new foundation in the valley of Absinthe, about half way between Dijon in France, and Geneva in Switzerland. The monks renamed the place, Clairvaux, "The Valley of Light." Less than fifty years later, at Bernard's death, the monastic order of Cistercians had so prospered that they grew exponentially, from three, to three hundred and forty three communities, spread throughout Europe.

A Supernatural Superabundance

Near the end of his life, Bernard wrote of his personal experience of God's transforming grace. The metaphor for which he is most famous is "the Kiss of the Bridegroom," taken from Solomon's *Song of Songs*. Let the reader mark the following: Bernard states and re-states that this "Kiss" was always *unfelt*. Nevertheless, he knew that the Lord was present, for

> as soon as He has entered into me, He has quickened my sleeping soul, has aroused and softened and goaded my heart, which was in a state of torpor and hard as stone. He has begun to pluck up and destroy, to plant and to build, to water the dry places, to illuminate the gloomy spots, to throw open those which were shut close, to inflame with warmth those

[places] which were cold, and to straighten its crooked paths and make its rough places smooth, so that my soul might bless the Lord and all that is within me praise His Holy name.[4]

Bernard preached eighty-six sermons on the first three chapters of the *Song of Songs*. The sermon series is incomplete; he died before he got any further. Like Augustine before him, Bernard testifies to prevenient grace, for he knows experientially that the love, the mercy and the kindnesses that he has received from God so freely poured out without measure, come only as gift. He titles his eighty-fourth sermon, *"The soul, seeking God, is anticipated by Him,"* and in it, he speaks of the ongoing call, and the ever-fuller revelation of grace that God purposes for us. In terms of the awakening of faith, Bernard speaks as an intimate lover and friend:

I do not think that when a soul has found Him, it will cease from seeking. God is sought, not by the movement of the feet, but by the desires of the heart; and when a soul has been so happy as to find Him, that sacred desire is not extinguished, but, on the contrary, is

[4] *Canticle 74.5,* quoted in Dom Cuthbert Butler, *Western Mysticism – Augustine, Gregory and Bernard.* Constable and Company, London, 1922, p.147.

increased. Is the consummation of the joy the extinction of the desire? It is rather to it as oil poured upon a flame; for desire is, as it were, a flame. Our joy will be fulfilled; but the fulfillment will not be the ending of the desire, nor therefore of the seeking.... Every soul among you that is seeking God should know that it has been anticipated by Him, and has been sought by Him before it began to seek Him. [5]

The apostle admonished Timothy, to "do the work of an evangelist."[6] In this present season of grace, it is clearer than ever before that we are not the ones initiating. As we seek to share faith with the unsaved, we do well to remind ourselves of Bernard's counsel: "Every soul that is seeking God ... has been anticipated by Him, and has been sought by Him before it began to seek Him;" especially since issues of pride, control, insecurity, and drivenness can so easily rise up and corrupt our best intentions. Any time we attempt to accomplish any work of the Kingdom, especially evangelism, the Lord's words need to be ringing in our ears: "Apart from Me you can do nothing."[7] It is His initiative, and not ours, that draws the unsaved.

[5] *Late Medieval Mysticism,* ed. Ray Petry. Library of Christian Classics, Westminster Press, Philadelphia, 1957, p.74.
[6] 2 Timothy 4.5.
[7] John 15.5.

"Belch Forth of thy Fullness"

Bernard of Clairvaux continues to serve as a helpful resource, for in a sermon written for Pentecost Sunday, he takes up the image of new wine.

Speaking of experiences so very similar to many who have found themselves "Toronto Blessed," he works things further, and marks the progress of the digestive process:

> It is [in] prayer that we drink the wine of the Spirit, which intoxicates the soul with holy love.... This wine irrigates the parched interior of the heart, facilitates the digestion of the meat of good works, and distributes the nutriment amongst the members of the soul (if you allow me the expression), confirming faith, fortifying hope, enlivening and regulating charity, and anointing all our actions with the rich unction of grace.

Changing metaphors, he continues:

> My brethren, if you be wise, you will make yourselves to be reservoirs rather than conduits. The difference between a conduit and a reservoir is this, that whereas the former discharges all its waters almost as soon as it is received, the latter waits until it is full to the brim, and only communicates what is

superfluous, what it can give away without loss to itself.

As spiritual father, Bernard takes the liberty to speak correction to those who are so keen to pour out their lives:

> We have in the Church today many conduits and but very few reservoirs. So great is the charity of those through whom the celestial streams of knowledge are communicated to us, that they want to give away before they have received. They are more willing to speak than to listen. They are forward to teach what they have not learned. Although unable to govern themselves, they gladly undertake to rule others. Thy charity is either non-existent, or so delicate and reed-like that it bends to every blast.

He names the internal conflict of high and noble aspirations of loving neighbour even more than self, while at the same time being so spiritually unstable that one "dissolves in consolation, faints under fear, loses its peace in sadness, is contracted by greed, distracted by ambition, disquieted by suspicion, disturbed by reproof, tormented with care, inflated with honour, consumed with envy." He calls his brothers to a posture of spiritual stability:

My brothers, learn to belch forth of thy fullness, and do not desire to be more generous than God.... The charity which combines prudence with generosity is wont to flow in before flowing out.... Behold now how much has to be poured into us in order that we may venture to pour out, giving of our plenitude, not of our poverty.[8]

* * *

Around the world, there are those who have grown impatient, even criticizing the repeated coming forward for prayer that characterizes renewal ministry. "How much 'carpet time' does one need before one gets down to business?" With the journalist who wrote the piece quoted from the *Island Herald* in Chapter One, there are many who are highly committed to answer our Lord's clear call to Kingdom ministry, especially when they are passionately concerned about the lostness of the lost, and the need for Gospel justice and righteousness within our political and social systems. It is asked repeatedly of the "Toronto Blessing," "Where's the fruit of all of this?" With the Apostle Paul, many answer relationally: we will keep coming forward for prayer until "we know the height and depth, the

---

[8] *St. Bernard's Sermons for the Seasons and Principal Festivals of the Year, vol.II.* Browne and Nolan, Dublin, 1923, pgs. 176-183.

length and breadth of the love of Christ, and to know it, though it is beyond knowledge."[9]

In terms of ministry, many of us have recognized that we have lived and attempted to minister, as Bernard put it, as conduits rather than reservoirs. We have more than realized that our attempts to serve only as conduits of grace so quickly leave us barren and empty, with no resources but our own abilities and best intentions as hollow shells.

Our spirits are being renewed and revived as the Lord so mercifully pours out His Spirit upon us, and we are finding that as we continue to rest in His love, ever looking to His grace for a fuller and fuller filling, the reservoirs of the Spirit are full and overflowing, and not just with a superabundance, but a supernatural superabundance. Instead of flesh giving birth to flesh, Spirit is birthing spirit. And in terms of evangelism, there are so many who have such wonderful testimonies of the glorious overflow of grace from their lives. Carla Doyle is one of them.

Over the Top

Carla came to the renewal meetings in Melbourne, Florida, early in 1995. Without apology, she came in desperation, and freely received grace upon grace. She was physically ill with severe back problems (severe spinal arthritis and advanced osteoporosis) which had

[9] Ephesians 3.19.

put her on a disability allowance for over six years. Several weeks before her first meeting, Carla had been widowed; several weeks before her husband's death, she had adopted her two pre-teen grandsons – her daughter is a cocaine addict, and her son-in-law had committed suicide. Not surprisingly, her grandsons had been under psychiatric care and on medication for four years due to the trauma of their life circumstances.

As the Tabernacle hosted renewal meetings six nights a week, Carla estimates that she came over one hundred and twenty times that first year, responding to every call for prayer ministry, "soaking herself" in the love of her Father, and allowing the Spirit to heal more and more of her heart. She committed herself completely to God, and asked Him to make her and the boys whole. She then told Him that she wanted to be His vessel in any way He chose.

Gently, yet systematically, God began to work in her life and the lives of her boys. For 30 years, Carla was chemically dependent on prescribed anti-depressants, but no longer. Both her grandsons no longer need their medications, nor the psychiatric care. The pain and physical immobility of Carla's back problems have nearly disappeared.

In March of 1996, this fifty-six year old grandmother and her eight and nine year old boys left for five months of training and field duty with Mercy Ships International. After three months of schooling, they spent two months in Puerto Cabezas, Nicaragua, where

Carla was asked to co-ordinate local evangelism. She served five different church denominations, several schools, an orphanage, a prison, as well as a street ministry. She and her team did everything from well drilling, to teaching personal hygiene; they refurbished a children's playground, and prayed for dying children. They had the privilege of seeing people come to the Lord through their personal witnessing.

At the conclusion of her field training, Carla returned home. She is furthering her studies, and is worshipping with her home church. These are her concluding remarks:

> "I have returned to Renewal here at the Tabernacle in anticipation of what God will show me through this ministry. I pray for more of God's anointing and the opportunity to minister to others with what He's already given me. But most of all, I pray to once again exalt Him on the mission field."

* * *

Learning to See

Obviously, not all of us are called to the nations. But this present outpouring of God's Spirit *is* preparing His Church for the end-time harvest, whenever the Lord sovereignly calls it in. That *is* the eschatological horizon towards which we are moving.

Wherever the Lord has us, with whomever the Lord has us, the salvation of the lost is His heart's desire. It is ours to have compassion on the next one. Here, we have a wonderful freedom, for we know that God's lovingkindness goes before us. As we meet with friends and strangers, we call forth one of the distinctives of grace based evangelism, discernment.

It is as if we each have a window to our spirits. And it is only spiritual discernment that enables us to perceive how wide open the window of faith is in a particular individual. If it is closed, it does not serve to smash it in, or to try to pry it open. Again and again in the Gospels, most of the Pharisees were closed, locked and barred; Nicodemus was an exception. Further, the rich young ruler walked away *from Jesus*. His window was boarded over by materialism.

There were times, however, when the pendulum was swung to the other extreme. The centurion from Capernaum threw his window wide open: "...only say the word...." Jesus remarks: "Not even in Israel have I found such faith."[10]

Evangelism is by its very nature a supernatural work. As we have compassion on the next one, we are also asking continuously, "How are You at work here Father? What have You orchestrated for this encounter, this moment?" As we seek to discern what it is the Lord has purposed, we recognize that it is not so much the

[10] Luke 7.7-9.

189

case that we have to "do or say something." Rather, we *search our hearts*. We search our hearts for the love that our Heavenly Father has for the person we are with. Here the heart leads, and the mind serves. Is there love reaching out, and love being revealed? Or is our motive for involvement driven by performance? Are we seeking to impress someone? Is it an issue of spiritual ego or superiority? Or, do we quickly and continuously remember our grounding in grace, and pray for a further measure of compassion and mercy?

Spiritual gifts and grace flow through love inspired by the Spirit, not through technique and methodology. In the Gospels, we read repeatedly that "His heart went out to them." "He had compassion on them...."[11]

* * *

Radical Abandon

This much is safe. The dynamics at work in the "Toronto Blessing" have stretched most of us, such that we recognize that far more is at work in this day. Many were taken far beyond their proverbial comfort zones during the second anniversary week at the Toronto Airport Christian Fellowship, for which over three thousand believers had gathered. One evening, Paul Cain was preaching. Paul can be considered one of our

---

[11] Matthew 9.36; 14.14; 15.32; 20.34; Mark 1.41; 6.34; 8.2; Luke 7.13; cf. Luke 15.20, the prodigal's father.

190

generation's prophetic grandfathers. He is a senior statesman for the Body of Christ; it was a high privilege to have him take part in our anniversary celebrations.

His message that particular night was titled, "Dignity or the Anointing." Early into the sermon, a gentleman in the second row started "Oh-ing." He got louder and louder. John Arnott looked in his direction, smiled, and told the surrounding ministry team to soak him. As they prayed, he manifested more and more boisterously. He was soon on the floor; not long thereafter, he had crawled underneath the front row of chairs, and was in the open ministry area, now "praying" for those resting in the Spirit. Over one man in particular, he was violently pounding judo chops into his chest, and yelling, "Release, release, release!!!"

The commotion was such that Paul was flustered; several of the three thousand people were on their feet, trying to see what was going on. I was seated only a few seats from the action, and thought repeatedly, "Why doesn't John have some of the ministry team take this guy to the back, and let them pray for him there?"

A few days later, I asked John that very question. His answer left me speechless. He said, "I know that man; I know his heart. I know how much he loves God, and how he has committed his life to follow and serve the Lord. I have no question as to his character. Once I know that, I don't care if it's Paul Cain, or three thousand people from all over the world that get offended. If the Spirit of God chooses to move on him there and then, I'm not going to offend the Holy Spirit. All I'm going to say is, 'More Lord.' "

The Question

Where is all of this going? Again, ultimately God pours out His Spirit for end-time harvest. That doesn't mean that twos and threes will be added to our churches on a given Sunday. It doesn't mean that twenty or thirty new believers will be added in a single week. Like the early Church, we may well see three thousand come to the Lord in a given day.

We quickly recognize that most local churches would be completely overwhelmed were that to happen. If, in a given week, the Lord added twenty newly converted pagans to our fellowships, many of us would be swamped. Especially if those twenty each reached one other unsaved friend the following week. We would then have forty newly saved, but as yet, undiscipled believers who radically change our status quo. They would be sitting in *our* seats, parking in our spots; it may well be that their kid pops our kid on the nose in Sunday school.

These new converts, however, are on fire for the Lord. The first twenty each reached two unsaved friends the next week, and the second twenty each shared faith with one other friend; the attendance the third week then swells to a total of one hundred new believers. The fourth week, in the favour of end-time harvest, doors and windows of faith might well be swung wide open, and those first twenty might each lead three others to Christ. The second twenty could lead two each; the third sixty, just getting started, would each lead one. That would mean that the net conversion growth for the four weeks amounted to two hundred and sixty new believers. These new believers would out-number the vast majority of existing church fellowships, all in the space of a month. If this growth track slowed, and merely doubled over the course of the next month, the church would have swelled to over four thousand – *but not into what was.*

This kind of growth will only be assimilated by a church that is completely dependent, completely yielded, completely attentive, and completely abandoned to and unashamed of whatever the Spirit calls forth, wherever, and whenever the Lord calls. That is why John Arnott's anniversary response so humbled me. I had never seen someone live out that kind of abandon before.

A Wing and a Prayer

One night, one of the Toronto Airport Christian Fellowship's ministry team, Lynn Patch, discovered how dynamic this radical obedience can be. After her small group fellowship meeting, Lynn felt hungry. It was about midnight, and though she does not usually eat late, she drove around till she found a pizza restaurant. All she wanted was a few chicken wings; the smallest order she was allowed to place included potato wedges, which she didn't want. While she waited for her order, she turned her back on the three East Indian men working behind the counter. She found herself praying, "Lord, what am I doing here? I'm not even hungry anymore." In the reflection of the store window, she saw herself, and the three men, standing behind her. Suddenly she knew why she was there. She turned around, and asked, "Do you guys know Jesus Christ?"

She did not expect their response. One of the men was pushed to the front. "He left India to come looking for Jesus! Your Jesus sent you here – tell him about your Jesus!"

Lynn began telling all three of them about the Lord, the only God. She shared the Gospel with them, and when she finished, Rajah, the man pushed forward, said that he believed that Jesus is God. He believed that because Jesus had come to him in a repeated dream. He knew it was Jesus because he had seen "pictures" of the Lord.

Rajah was so moved by these recurring dreams that he had tried to attend a Christian church in India. His father, however, forbade him to do so. Rajah was a successful lawyer in his 30's, but still lived at home. As he was under his father's authority, he was told in no uncertain terms that he would no longer be his son if he ever believed in Jesus.

Rajah not only left home; he left India, in order to find Jesus. He chose as his destination the city of Toronto, though he knew no one there. A Punjabi taxi driver took him to a local Sikh temple, where he met a man who gave him a job in the pizza restaurant.

This desperate man went to several Christian churches in his area, but no one ever spoke to him. The preachers gave no altar calls, and he did not feel secure enough to ask anyone about Jesus. He had been in Canada nearly a year when Lynn met him that night.

She led him through the sinner's prayer, and assured him of God's love. Rajah came to several meetings at the Toronto Airport Christian Fellowship with her, and began to be discipled. Shortly thereafter, he had to move into the heart of the city. There he began attending a local church.

* * *

If we are to respond to the works of amazing grace that the Lord purposes and orchestrates, a radical humility is called forth. As living sacrifices, our personal respectability, reputation, and control will most certainly have to be laid down. Together with the apostle Paul, we may find ourselves as "fools for Christ," assured only in the knowledge that the "folly of God is wiser than human wisdom."[12]

This is one of the reasons why there really is only one

---

[12] Paul speaks at length along these lines in 1 Corinthians 1.18-4.21. He is speaking of the message of the cross, and his apostolic calling to preach Jesus, before whom there can be no human pride. (1.29).

of two responses to this outpouring of God's Spirit: either one finds release, or offence. After a brief time for investigation and discernment, one must conclude either "Toronto Blessing" or "Toronto Blasphemy." There really is no middle ground. Those who speak of the Toronto *"Experience"* are noncommittally "Laodicean."[13] To conclude "it's God, but we don't want it" is anathema.

The Way Ahead

Those "in," however, find themselves continuously stretched. Some of us have recognized that when we are offended, we need to get used to it. As never before, we have learned that the Lord's question in Isaiah 43.19 is a rhetorical one: "See, I am doing a new thing; now it springs up – can you not perceive it?" The appropriate answer? "No, Lord, we do not understand. Not quite yet, Lord. Please show us more."

We can glean further revelation from one of the minor prophets, Zechariah. His name means "the Lord remembers," and he writes to encourage the captives returning from Babylon. Many of his prophecies foretold the coming of the Messiah – the King meekly riding on a donkey; the good shepherd sold for thirty pieces of silver; the pierced one beheld; the One at whose death the sheep are scattered.[14] There are also

---

[13] See Revelation 3.14-22.
[14] Zechariah 9.9 and Matthew 21.9; Zechariah 11.12 and Matthew

several prophecies that anticipate and describe the second coming of the Lord – the four horsemen, the measuring of the holy city, and the two olive trees and lampstands.[15]

Chapter 14 tells of the day when "the Lord will go out and fight against the nation, fighting as on a day of battle." Two verses later, the Lord is attended by all the holy ones, and in verse 9, His majesty and dominion is declared: "The Lord will become King over all the earth; on that day He will be the only Lord and His name the only name."

The tenth chapter of Zechariah is a bridge between the first and second coming of the Lord. The text foretells God's victorious triumph over His foes; twenty-six times, there is the future description of what the Lord "will" do, what His people "will" be like, what destiny "will" come to pass. In this season of blessing, as we attend to where all of this is going, these verses are particularly suggestive.

In verse one, God's people are told to "ask the Lord for rain at the time of the spring rain, the Lord who makes the storm clouds." At the outset, it is imperative that we recognize, yet again, that it is the Lord, and the Lord alone, who is the One taking the initiative. We

---

26.15; Zechariah 12.10 and John 19.37; Zechariah 13.7 and Matthew 26.31.

[15] Zechariah 1.7f. and Revelation 6.1f.; Zechariah 1.16 and Revelation 11.1-2; Zechariah 4.11-14 and Revelation 11.4-10.

cannot make it rain. We cannot fabricate the storm clouds. Once it is raining, however, we are invited to ask for *more*. Grace is again on the forefront. We ask for more, and the Lord promises that He will give the heavy rains, unto abundant harvest.

Radical Transformation

The third verse begins with the declaration of God's anger over the faithlessness of His shepherds and leaders. What follows is the promise that He Himself will extend care to His flock. In the latter part of the verse, there is a most unusual metaphor – the Lord's flock will be "transformed into war horses." Regrettably, the NIV translation diminishes this dynamic: [the Lord will] "make them a proud horse in battle." One can only wonder what has to take place to turn a cuddly little sheep into a war horse! Tongue in cheek, there will most likely be those who complain that it does not happen "decently and in order."

However one envisions becoming a war horse, Zechariah keeps his readers reeling. Four verses later, he uses another striking metaphor: God raises up an outrageous army, "with hearts gladdened *as if* with wine." Across the page, in Chapter 9.15, this same army is described as being "roaring drunk *as if* with wine."

Before my conversion, I had a practised knowledge of what it was to be roaring drunk with wine. That part of the picture is not a puzzle. The "as if" bit is. Why would the Lord want His army to be roaring drunk, as if with wine? Without praising alcoholic drunkenness in any way, there are a few observations that may shed some light on this peculiar text. When one is drunk, there is not much by way of striving. One's task drivenness is suppressed. "Time to go? What's your rush? Have another drink...." Further, one's inhibitions are characteristically loosened. There comes a false sense of freedom, even license; boundaries and limits fall. That is one of the reasons driving while drunk is so dangerous. A final observation: some find that while drunk, they are not nearly so intimidated. That's why beer brawls are so common.

In the Spirit, God purposes to raise up His army. These are a people who are militant, but not full of themselves. There is no striving, and neither intimidation nor inhibition. The Lord's army is not bound by limitations, for the Lord Himself is with them. It is in this context that we understand an earlier verse, Zechariah 4.6 "...not by might, nor by power, but by My Spirit says the Lord." The Lord's army is overcome, not with wine, but with the Spirit of Jesus.

Again and again, it is declared that the Lord is the One leading. In verse 8 He says, "I shall whistle to call them in, for I have delivered them." A complementary verse may be found in Isaiah 5.26: "He will also lift up a standard to the distant nation, and will whistle for it from the ends of the earth; And behold, it will come with speed."

In this season of blessing, it is as if there is a catalytic acceleration to the work of God's grace right around the world. In terms of conversions, it is indeed as if the Lord has whistled, and with that clear call, the lost have found their way home. Gary Patton, of the Toronto Airport's New Life team, tells of one remarkable story.

A middle-aged Japanese businessman was facing bankruptcy in Japan. He was at his wits' end. Unexplainably, he sensed that he was to come to Canada. He contacted his travel agent, but never having been to Canada, he couldn't name a particular city as his destination. "Vancouver...? Toronto...? Montreal....?" asked his travel agent. Toronto sounded good to him.

He had no idea what he was doing, or why he was doing it. This gentleman was neither a Christian, nor a practising religious. He had never heard of the "Toronto Blessing." Once he had disembarked, he picked up his luggage, and cleared customs. Standing in the meeting area, he wondered an equivalent, "Now what?" He spoke no English.

A Japanese woman and her son were waiting for one of their family that had arrived on the same plane as the businessman. The woman felt that the Lord was telling her to go talk to this Japanese businessman, and she obeyed. As she heard his story, she had no doubt about this appointment; once they had met their family member, she took the businessman to their home. The next day, she brought him to her church's Sunday service. Her church is the Toronto Airport Christian Fellowship.

The woman's son translated for the businessman, and when the salvation call was given, the man wanted to respond. The boy came forward with him, in order to continue translating. The man accepted Jesus as his Saviour and Lord, and during his altar counselling, he received the baptism of the Spirit. (It was at this point that Gary was called in to answer a few questions.)

After hearing out the story, Gary asked the boy, "Why did you bring this man here?" The answer was simple enough: "'Cause he needed Jesus." After they prayed for the businessman some more, he walked away with a huge smile on his face, knowing EXACTLY why he was to come to Toronto. He returned to Japan the following day.

The Lord's War Horses

Many, if not most, Christians feel a sense of panic when they hear the word "evangelism." At one end of the spectrum, there are some who are chagrined at the thought of forcing one's religious opinions on another. "A spirit of tolerance and co-existence is what is needed at the close of the millennium." At the other end are those who feel a gnawing guilt because they have never led a single person to the Lord.

So much changes as God freely and abundantly fills us with His Spirit. In this present season of blessing, new measures of faith and faithfulness have been awakened, such that many are enabled to share the love of God with a new freedom, boldness and authority.

There has come the recognition that evangelism is not so much a task that *we* try to bring to conclusion, but rather, it is the work of *Christ*, in us and through us. Evangelism is by nature, supernatural!

Michael Green reflected on one of the reasons many of us have never spoken about our faith to others: we have felt too empty for the "overflow" that constitutes true evangelism. "Like tourists going through customs, we've had nothing to declare."[16] But as we have received blessing, we know as never before that God's amazing grace precedes us, undergirds us, and swirls behind us. In that knowledge, inhibitions are stripped away, such that nothing is held back. Timidity gives way to an abandoned response to the work of Christ in us, such that we seek to bring the lost into His allegiance, "by word and deed, by the power of signs and wonders, and by the power of the Holy Spirit."[17] I thought of the apostle's words when I heard the following testimony at a recent conference.

Leigh-Anne, September 1996

Leigh-Anne is nineteen years old. She has been a Christian for almost two and a half years and presently works with the physically challenged as a care aid. Because of her background, her identity has been guarded.

[16] *Evangelism Through the Local Church.* Nelson Publishers, Nashville, 1992, p.14.
[17] Romans 15.18-19.

Growing up, I was never close to my family. They were alcoholics and there was a lot of abuse in our house. My biological parents were divorced when I was two and my mother was soon living with the man who is currently my stepfather. He is also an alcoholic. I was a very unhappy little girl, and remember long periods of time when I refused to speak to anyone.

I began smoking and using drugs at a very young age. I wasn't trying to be rebellious; I just couldn't find any other way to live with the hurt and the anger I felt. When I was fifteen I left home to live life in "the big city," thinking I could make it on a grade nine education. It wasn't long before I ended up on the streets, confused, lost and badly addicted to drugs. It was then that I was placed in a number of foster homes, but they never worked out. I had no idea what love was, and the only thing I seemed capable of doing was hating.

When I turned sixteen, I was sent back to my home town to live with my mother. It was only a few months later that she packed her bags and moved three provinces away. Before she left she signed documents that relinquished her guardianship. She told me I was no longer her daughter.

Over the next year and a half, I was in more foster homes. I got involved with the occult, and some really dangerous people. Before long my life was being threatened. I tried the best I could to protect myself, but to no avail. No one could help me. I remember lying in my bed one night, saying out loud, "Okay, If you're there, God, I need you to help me because no one else can." I scolded myself for being so stupid as to think that God was real, and never told anyone of my first "prayer."

Almost a year later, I was back in the city, living on my own. My drug habit was still raging and I became even more heavily involved in the occult. I was sitting in a coffee shop late one night with a friend, and a stranger about our age approached us. He had long hair, earrings, and a dark trench coat. He seemed pretty cool. After the introductions, Dave began to tell us about Jesus. I gave him all the attitude I could muster. He responded, "God's telling me things about you and I bet I could give you a detailed account of your life." I dared him to try. He told me about things there was no way he could have known. I was amazed! Dave then said, "I also know the first time you cried out to God." At this point I was scared because I knew that if this young guy knew about that time almost a year ago, then God was real. I tried to bluff.

"That's a lie. I've never cried out to God!" He closed his eyes for a minute and said, "It was nine months and thirteen days ago." He was right. I remembered that day so clearly because I had been so scared. I went home and checked my journal – Dave was dead right –nine months, thirteen days ago. I remembered that he had told me to ask God to reveal Himself to me in a dream that night. I did as he had told me to do, and God sure made Himself known! I dreamt of a golden cross appearing in the clouds before me. I knew Jesus was real!

I then began to go to the same church that I presently attend. Because of my past, and the way I looked, I figured they'd kick me out. Instead, a complete stranger walked up to me, hugged me and said, "Welcome home."

Since that time, God has delivered me from drugs and alcohol and restored every physical side effect I got from drugs. He has taught me how to speak blessing instead of curses, and each day He softens my heart more and teaches me more about His perfect love. Maybe I didn't believe in God, but He believed in me. He's saved me from so much, time and time again, and I'm so thankful. He even helped me go back and finish high school! His mercies are new each day!

As I've walked with the Lord, He's filled a place of emptiness with an immense love for His people. Whether we know Him or not, we are all His children, and He desperately wants us to know Him. The more I love Jesus, the more I love His people and, in turn, the more desperately I want His children to know Him.

My friend Donna and I often go out for coffee after work. On the way to the coffee shop, we pray for a "divine appointment," a meeting with a stranger who doesn't know Jesus. We ask the Lord to interrupt our evening with whatever we can do for Him. We sit down and talk, go about our normal business, and wait for Jesus to arrange a meeting.

One night in particular, we were in the restaurant, and Jesus really drew our attention to our waitress. We began to pray for her, and Jesus showed me in a picture that she was bulimic. I struggled with talking to her about it but Donna encouraged me a lot. When our waitress came back, I made a beginning. "We were just praying for you and I believe the Lord just showed me that you're bulimic. Could we pray for you?" She became very defensive and rude, and denied that she had ever even considered doing anything so horrible to change her appearance. I was devastated. I thought I had made God look ridiculous. Ten minutes later, she came back to our table. She was crying, and explained how she had just been discharged from the hospital for bulimia. She was suicidal and had exhausted all avenues of help. She let us pray for her and Jesus came and touched her. PRAISE GOD!

About a year ago, our church did a conference in Golden, British Columbia. During the weekend, we did an outreach in the park. We gave out hamburgers and drinks, and met a lot of young people that afternoon. We invited them all to the evening meeting. They pointed to a young guy in black across the park and said, "Don't invite Shawn. He's a satanist." My first reaction? God LOVES satanists! I went over to invite him and he said that Tom, a guy from our band, had already invited him, and we could just leave him alone.

That night, I arrived late for the meeting. Worship had already started. As I walked up the church steps,

Shawn came running out in a panic. "Something's happening in there! I can feel it! As soon as I went in I started shaking. What's going on?!!" My friend Jen stayed with him while I went to get Tom to come and pray. After prayer and conversation, Shawn had become the newest member of our family in Christ! God had sovereignly drawn Shawn to Himself because He knew Shawn's heart. Jesus knows us better than we know ourselves and He will do whatever it takes to reach us.

In August of this year, our church held a renewal meeting in one of our local parks. They had asked a few people to share their testimonies and before long, it was my turn. As I spoke, Jesus filled me with so much love for people that I began to cry. He laid it on my heart to invite people up for prayer. Guess who responded? Not the most intelligent people, not the most gifted people, not the most spiritual people, but little children. They came running up to me, pulling at me, saying, "We want to get prayed for!" What a picture of the Lord's heart.

Recently, I was hanging out on Granville Street (skid row) in Vancouver, with a mercy ministry from another church. A young guy, John, came up to me and was basically laughing at me because I was a Christian. He seemed to be the mouthy tough guy of his group of friends. I said, "Hey, man. Can I pray for you?" He let me, thinking I was giving him more ammunition for his mockery. I began to pray that God would shine His light. Then I told him, "Ask Jesus if He loves you." He hesitated. "Go ahead, ask Him." He did, and Jesus responded. I can't say I know exactly how (that's between John and the Lord) but his face softened and tears began to stream down his face. John is now walking with the Lord and attending a local church.

I realize that my generation is not all that pleasant to look at, and we're not exactly kind or eloquent. But we have nothing left to hope in, nothing to believe in, and nothing to look forward to. Sexual and physical abuse, drug addiction and abortion are normal in our lives and we don't know how to live through it. So, we internalize it and become angry and bitter towards adults, government, and any type of authority figure. It's only because we are hurt and dying and overcome with hopelessness. So, who's going to love us? Who's going to believe in us and love us back to life?

I believe that God has big plans for my generation and that He's gifted us and called us to it. But the workers are few and not all of us have found the way to freedom yet. Do you realize that the reason why we have systems like foster homes and welfare is because the Church hasn't done its job? GOD BELIEVES IN US!!! Please, I implore you, let Him show you that.

I also know that God believes in His Church, and so do I. During this renewal movement, I have been blessed to see God work miracles in the Body. He is reconstructing cold and resentful hearts so that they can love again. He is pulling down walls of division and stereotypes, and dealing with hidden sin. He's giving

His Bride joy again, and consuming her with passion for her Groom, Jesus. I believe we are all called to witness to this world, but how can we if we don't have love. God's Spirit is moving and equipping His Church with more than enough love for this world, if only we are willing.

God loves all His people more than we could ever comprehend. If you ask God to use you, He will, because He knows what state this world is in. The days are short and the Lord desperately wants to restore His Church, that it might be effective in reaching an otherwise hopeless generation.

* * *

In Joel 2.28 and Acts 2.17, the Father's sovereign purpose is declared: "in the last days, says the Lord, I will pour out My Spirit on all mankind; sons and daughters shall prophesy, young men shall see visions, and old men shall dream dreams." The outpouring of His Spirit is to one end only: that "whosoever calls on the name of the Lord shall be saved."

Leigh-Anne's life and witness is a grace-filled demonstration of Joel 2/Acts 2. Through Spirit-initiated words, pictures, visions, and dreams, these prophetic stirrings and urgings move us to reach out with supernatural authority and freedom. In the power of the Spirit, we love, speak, and bless, confident that the Lord goes before us, opening doors, and initiating *kairos* moments, such that the lost find themselves found in the love of the Father.

Grace based evangelism is not so much a particular methodology to be learned, or a strategic program to be followed. But as has been demonstrated through all the testimonies, neither is it a totally passive "waiting on God" that keeps the Gospel unspoken. Again and again, the Spirit releases the authority and the grace for the Lord's witnesses to ask the noon-time questions: "Do you know Jesus? Would you like to?"

Part of me, however, remains frustrated, for there is a sense that I still do not know "how" to win the lost. It is not for lack of content. The following page and a half may serve those who do not know what to say when someone is ready to receive Christ.

While we must be able to tell someone the basics of the Gospel of Jesus Christ, it is not we who do the soul-winning. Rather, ours is the humble and surrendered recognition that salvation comes only as Jesus said it would: "No one can come to Me unless he is drawn by the Father."[18] In this, we are totally *dependent*, not totally passive. The Lord has called us as His witnesses, and in this season of blessing, we have so much *more* to declare. As we open our hearts to receive an ever greater revelation of our Father's love for us, we receive a graced impregnation that, when nurtured, yields fruitfulness.

[18] John 6.44.

All around us are divinely ordained moments of grace... and as we have compassion on the next one, and attend to what the Lord purposes in this particular moment, we will discover greater faith, and freedom, and ever more grace.

S.D.G.

FAITH SHARING

* * *

If we have compassion on the next one, and if we are attending to what the Spirit is calling forth in our midst, sooner or later, someone will say to us: "I've been watching you. There's something to this Christianity business. I want what you have. How do I become a Christian?" Alternatively, the Spirit will convince us that it is time to ask, "Do you know Jesus?"

The following may serve those who do not know what to say next.

In John's Gospel, Chapter 1, verse 10, we read, "He (Jesus) was in the world; but the world, though it owed its being to Him, did not recognize Him."

1. "Recognize."

When we strip Christian faith right down, the first thing we have to say is that being a Christian means recognizing Jesus. John puts it in the negative here – the world, the unbelieving world, did NOT recognize Jesus. When we turn that around, a believer, a follower of Jesus, DOES recognize Him.

What does it mean to recognize someone? It means

to know something about that person. You can't "recognize" a stranger.

In terms of recognizing Jesus, **what do we have to know about Him?** Remember, we are keeping this simple. What needs to be recognized in Jesus? Let me suggest this: Jesus is the **Son of God**, and the **Giver of Life**. We need to recognize that Jesus wants to change our lives. Jesus shows us what life is really meant to be like – what love, peace, joy, and freedom truly are. Stripped right down, we need to recognize that in Jesus, there is a **quality** to life, a **desirability** to life, that is missing without Him.

However, we can't stop there. It is quite possible to recognize that someone loves us, but be totally unmoved by that love. John 1.11 makes this very declaration: "He (Jesus) entered His own realm, and His own would not... receive Him."

2. "Receive."

Not only do we have to recognize Jesus; we have to receive His love. **We ask Jesus the Life-changer to change OUR lives**. What Jesus most changes in our lives is our sin, all that has mashed and marred our living. He takes all of that on Himself, dying in our place, so that we can know His sinless life, as He lives in us. He is willing to exchange His life for ours, because He loves each of us so much.

It doesn't stop there. In John 1.12 we read: "To all who did receive Him, to those who believed in His name, He gave the right to become children of God."

3. "Believed in His name." To recognize and receive Jesus is not enough. There is a personal response called forth. Recognition and reception of Jesus re-orients our lives such that we live under a new "name," a new authority. Most of us have trouble with authority; we don't like being told what to do, even if our best interests are on the line. That's one of the reasons many people never "believe in the name of Jesus."

What does "believing in His name" mean for our daily lives? It means that we decide to **name Christ as THE authority in our lives**. Maybe we hold our hands open, as a symbol of our abandonment to Him; maybe **we simply say "Yes, Lord."** Then, as the Spirit of Jesus lives in us, He shows us what that "Yes, Lord" involves.

1. **Recognizing Jesus**, and wanting the life He has to give.
2. **Receiving Jesus**, and accepting the love He brings to our lives.
3. **Believing in the name of Jesus**, and allowing His Spirit to transform our lives, saying our "Yes" to what He wills for us.

Bob George puts it all in one sentence: "Jesus Christ laid down His life *for us*, so that He could give His life *to us*, so that He could live His life *through us*."[1]

---

[1] *Basic Christianity.* Harvest House Publishers, Eugene, Oregon, 1989, p.174.

BIBLIOGRAPHY

Augustine. *Confessions*. trans. J.G. Pilkerton. Nicene
and Post Nicene Fathers, First Series, vol. 1.
Peabody, Massachusetts: Hendrickson
Publishers,1994.

Evans, Eivion. *The Welsh Revival of 1904*.
Worcester: Evangelical Press of Wales, 1969.

Green, Michael. *Evangelism through the Local
Church*. Nashville: Thomas Nelson, Pub., 1992.

Jones, Brynmor Pierce. *An Instrument of Revival: The
Complete Life of Evan Roberts*. South Plainfield,
N.J.: Bridge Publishing, 1995.

_____. *Voices From the Welsh Revival 1904-
1905*. Bridgend: Evangelical Press of Wales, 1995.

Lloyd- Jones, Martin. *Revival*. Wheaton, Illinois:
Crossway Books, 1987.

McGavran, Donald. *Understanding Church Growth, 3rd. ed.* Grand Rapids, Michigan: William B. Eerdmans Pub. Co., 1990.

The Revival of Religion: Addresses by Scottish Evangelical Leaders. Edinburgh: The Banner of Truth Trust, 1840/1984.

Synan, Vincent, ed. *Aspects of Pentecostal-Charismatic Origins.* Plainfield, N.J.: Logos International, 1975.

推推小手
祛百病

张振宇◎主 编　　袁 娜　王成远◎副主编

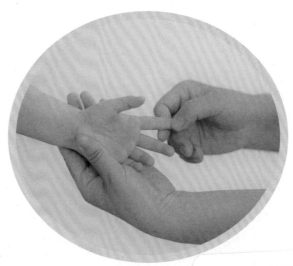

中国人口出版社
China Population Publishing House
全国百佳出版单位

图书在版编目（CIP）数据

推推小手祛百病 / 张振宇主编 . -- 北京 : 中国人
口出版社 , 2021.1
ISBN 978-7-5101-7190-1

Ⅰ. ①推… Ⅱ. ①张… Ⅲ. ①小儿疾病—按摩疗法 (
中医) Ⅳ. ① R244.1

中国版本图书馆 CIP 数据核字 (2020) 第 195135 号

推推小手祛百病
TUITUI XIAOSHOU QU BAIBING

张振宇　主编

责 任 编 辑	李玉景	
责 任 印 制	林　鑫　单爱军	
装 帧 设 计	北京品艺文化传播有限公司	
出 版 发 行	中国人口出版社	
印　　　刷	和谐彩艺印刷科技（北京）有限公司	
开　　　本	710 毫米 × 1000 毫米	1/16
印　　　张	8	
字　　　数	130 千字	
版　　　次	2021 年 1 月第 1 版	
印　　　次	2021 年 1 月第 1 次印刷	
书　　　号	ISBN 978-7-5101-7190-1	
定　　　价	36.80 元	

网　　　址	www.rkcbs.com.cn
电 子 信 箱	rkcbs@126.com
总编室电话	（010）83519392
发行部电话	（010）83510481
传　　　真	（010）83538190
地　　　址	北京市西城区广安门南街 80 号中加大厦
邮 政 编 码	100054

前　言

　　作为家长，最关心的就是孩子的健康。每当孩子感冒、发热、咳嗽、呕吐的时候，父母都非常揪心。但小孩子"脏腑娇嫩，形气未充"，身体发育尚未完善，非常容易生病，而且小儿是"纯阳之体"，受到病邪侵害时，容易从阳化热，引起发热等病症。一旦孩子生病，家长往往一筹莫展，除了上医院，似乎没有别的办法。

　　小儿推拿是祖先留下来的宝贵遗产，孩子的小手更是开启这个宝藏的关键！孩子的五根手指对应着五脏的经络，关乎心、肝、脾、肺、肾等的健康，孩子的手臂上藏着清火、退热的要穴。了解孩子小手上的秘密，平时给他做一做保健按摩，当孩子生小病时进行对症按摩，孩子的健康就会牢牢掌握在父母手中。

　　当孩子出现积食、发热、咳嗽、呕吐、咽痛等小病症时，只要按照书中的方法，推一推、揉一揉孩子小手上的穴位，你会发现，孩子的症状很快就会减轻，坚持按摩几天，孩子多半就康复了。当然，并不是说孩子有病就不用去医院了，遇到家长自己拿不准的情况还是需要及时就诊，以免贻误病情。

　　为了让家长朋友能够掌握小儿推拿的基本知识，让孩子少生病，少去医院，健康成长，我们根据自己的临床经验并查阅相关文献，编写了此书，希望本书能成为家长育儿的枕边书，随时随地学习起来，为孩子的健康保驾护航。

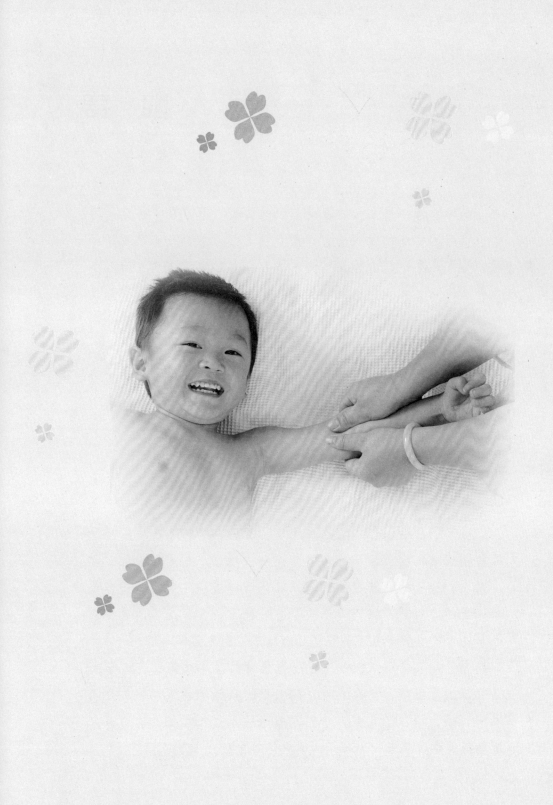

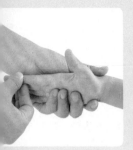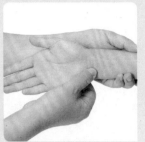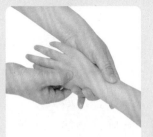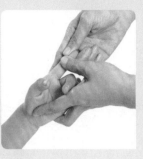

目 录

01　小儿推拿，父母一定要掌握的技能

02　小手上的 20 个特效穴位

03　推拿治疗 15 种小儿常见病

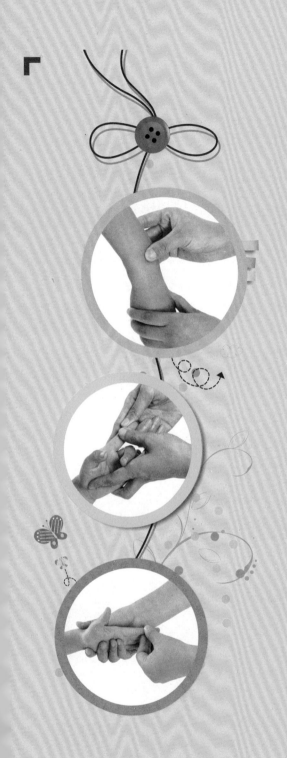

01

小儿推拿，父母一定要掌握的技能

孩子的双手就是一座随身携带的医药宝库

小儿推拿是以中医理论为指导，应用手法于穴位，作用于小儿机体，以调整脏腑、经络、气血功能，从而达到防病治病目的的一种技术。小儿推拿有着悠久的历史，近年来也得到广泛的认可和推广。

孩子具有独特的体质、五脏特点，每个年龄段也有着不同的养育特点，所以孩子的经络、穴位与成年人有所不同。特别是小儿手部穴位更是小儿独有的医药宝库，在15岁之前，这些穴位都具有明显的功效。推拿孩子的小手就能达到治病防病的目的，原因有以下几点：

第一，双手是阳气之本，推双手可提升阳气。

小儿的身体非常娇嫩，五脏还没有发育完全。五脏虚弱，外邪易入侵，很容易生病。《黄帝内经》中明确指出"四肢者，诸阳之本也"，以及"邪布于四末"。四肢是阳气的根本。所以，通过小儿手部推拿，可以激发阳气，使阴阳平衡，从而达到治病防病的目的。现代医学也认为，四肢是人体的末梢，它是最敏感的，稍一受到刺激，全身就会有反应。所以，当身体生病的时候，就可以通过刺激身体末梢来治病。

第二，小儿手部的穴位更加敏感。

成年人身体上的穴位，可以说是"一个萝卜一个坑"，一个点就是一个穴位。但是，中医的先贤们发现，孩子的手掌比较小，所以穴位不是呈点状，而是呈线状或片状。更重要的是，孩子小手上有很多特定的穴位，长大后这些穴位就不敏感了。就像小儿腹泻、呕吐，只要推一推孩子胃经，即拇指掌面第一节，就可以很快缓解症状；而当孩子出现胸闷、咳喘时，就可以推一推孩子的无名指螺纹面，即孩子的肺经，以缓解症状。

第三，小儿手部穴位起效更快。

实践发现，当孩子生病时，推拿孩子手部（上肢）穴位起效非常迅速。比如小儿发热，推拿天河水300～500次，能迅速退烧。虽然四肢都有穴位，孩子的双足和双手一样，都可以治病，但是两手的效果更好。父母学习并掌握小儿双手推拿的穴位

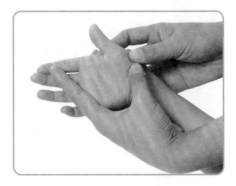

及手法，就可以提升小儿身体里的阳气，促进阴阳平衡，保障孩子的身体健康。

小儿百脉，汇于两掌

与成年人穴位的分布具有最大区别的就是孩子小手（上肢）穴位了，这是小儿所独有的，也是最为神奇的。孩子小手的五根手指，对应着脾经、胃经、肝经、心经、肺经、肾经。孩子五指上的经络通过不同的排列组合，就可以辅助治疗各种疾病，再配以最合适的按摩手法和力度，就能发挥出令人惊叹的魔力。

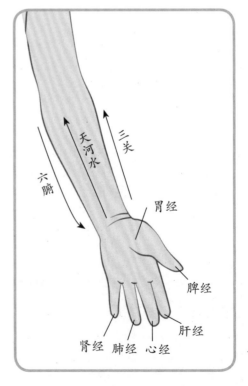

◆拇指：对应脾经和胃经

婴幼儿脾常不足，经常出现食欲不振、消化不良、疳积、腹泻、

咳嗽、消瘦等症。父母经常给孩子推推拇指外侧缘或拇指掌面近掌端第一节，能增强孩子食欲。长期坚持，孩子就会摆脱消化不良、消瘦、疳积等造成的困扰，身体逐渐强壮起来。

◆食指：对应肝经

肝藏血，一般情况下，肝虚的孩子很容易盗汗和抽筋。父母平时如果经常给孩子推推食指末节螺纹面，即肝经，对盗汗和抽筋有一定的治疗效果。

◆中指：对应心经

如果孩子老是心神不安、一惊一乍或爱出虚汗，则属于心虚；若孩子面红发热、长口疮、小便短赤或心烦不安，则属于心热。以上病症，都应该从心治，推孩子的中指末节螺纹面，即心经，对孩子的这些病症都有很好的疗效。

◆无名指：对应肺经

如果孩子的声音很弱，说话总是没底气，那就有可能是肺虚；如果孩子总是发不出声音或者嗓音经常变得嘶哑，则有可能表示肺里有痰；如果孩子总浑身无故发痒，则有可能是肺燥。父母可以经常给孩子推无名指螺纹面来缓解以上不适。

◆小指：对应肾经

孩子的遗尿、流口水等问题，都应该与肾脏有一定的关系。父母可以经常推推孩子的小指末节螺纹面，即肾经部位。

此外，孩子前臂掌侧正中那条线是天河水，清天河水可以清孩子体内的热毒，对热证有疗效。手臂桡侧靠拇指的那条线是三关，体弱多病的孩子适合推三关，可以补充气血，让孩子强壮起来。手臂尺侧靠小指的那条线是六腑，退六腑清热凉血，能够去除孩子体内的实热大毒。

如何让孩子接受并适应经络按摩

　　小儿推拿的最佳对象是5岁以下的孩子，婴幼儿尤为适宜。但临床治疗的患者中，年龄在15岁以下的孩子还占相当一部分。

　　父母应该尽早学习和掌握小儿推拿的方法，从孩子一出生，就每天给他做保健性的按摩、亲子抚触，开启孩子自身的宝藏，提高其免疫力和自愈力。只要每天坚持做，孩子也会养成习惯，避免在他长大一些后因为不适应、不接受，或者怕疼、怕痒等，使按摩无法进行。

　　有些孩子比较敏感，进行推拿的时候，会有抵触心理，家长要耐心给孩子做示范，刚开始不要急于求成。可以像做游戏一样跟孩子玩，跟孩子一起对着图片找穴位，让孩子也给父母揉一揉、按一按，在亲子互动中，让孩子自然而然地接受推拿按摩。长此以往，孩子不光会喜欢上按摩，说不定还会"上瘾"呢！睡前给孩子揉一揉肚子，推一推攒竹，按一按眼周，揉一揉耳朵，孩子会非常安心地睡去，睡眠质量也很高。

　　每天给孩子做保健按摩，也会成为非常美好的亲子时光。父母温暖的手带给孩子的不仅是健康，更多的是爱。经常被父母爱抚的孩子心理上会更有安全感，这对身体发育、智力发育都非常有益。

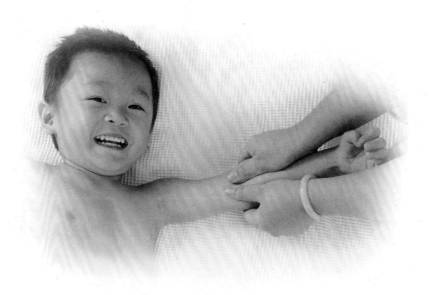

小儿按摩有顺序，按摩频次要讲究

　　小儿推拿操作应按一定顺序进行，临床上有三种方法。一是先头面，次上肢，再胸腹、腰背，最后是下肢；二是先推主穴，后推配穴；三是先推配穴，后推主穴。

　　推拿的先后顺序可根据病情轻重缓急或小儿体位而定。如脾虚腹泻可先推上肢主穴，补大肠经，后推腰背部配穴，推上七节骨；胃热呕吐，则可先推上肢配穴清板门，清大肠经，最后推颈项部主穴天柱骨。治疗时可根据小儿机体情况灵活掌握。如哭闹的小儿已熟睡，则可先摩腹，以免小儿醒时哭闹，腹肌紧张，影响治疗效果。

　　小儿推拿手法操作的时间，应根据孩子年龄的大小、体质的强弱、疾病的轻重缓急，以及手法的特性等因素而定。治疗频率通常每日1次，高热等急性热病可每日2次，慢性病可隔日1次。治疗的时间每次10～15分钟，一般不超过20分钟，也可根据具体情况灵活掌握。

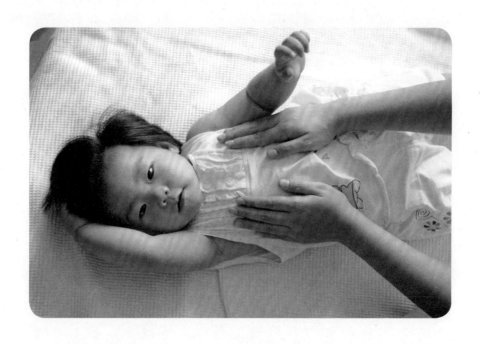

适当的推拿次数和频率能使疾病很快痊愈；相反，推拿次数少、时间短，达不到治疗量，就达不到治疗效果。但是也应注意，次数过多、频率过快对孩子身体无益，反而有害。对年龄大、体质强、病属实证的孩子，操作次数可以多一些，频率可以快一些；对于年龄小、体质弱、病属虚证的孩子则相对次数少一些，频率慢一些。一般1岁的孩子，使用推、揉、摩、运等较柔和的手法操作，一个穴位推300下左右。小儿年龄大、体质强、疾病重，主穴可多推些；年龄小、身体弱，配穴要少推些。一般小儿推拿采用掐、按、拿、搓、摇等手法，只需3～5次即可。

按摩方向很关键

小儿推拿穴位除常用的十四经穴、经外奇穴与成年人相似外，大多数为小儿特定穴位。这些穴位呈点、线、面状，多分布在两肘以下和头面部，以两手居多。推拿特定穴是小儿经络按摩的特点之一，这些穴位以特定的操作方向决定补泻性质。根据穴区点、线、面状分布的规律，手法操作分为直线方向和旋转方向两种。

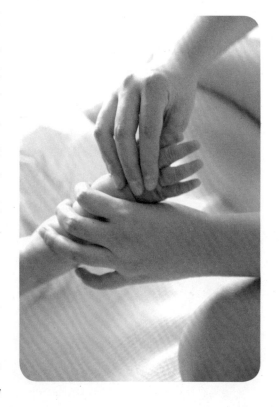

直线方向的操作，主要用推法。如分布在手掌的脾经、胃经、肝经、心经、肺经等，其补泻方向大体相同，即向指尖推为泻，向指根推为补。但肾经与之相反。有些非特定穴在经络线上，如中

脘、三阴交等，它们共同的补泻规律是顺经络走行方向推为补，逆经络走行方向推为泻，来回顺逆方向推属平补平泻。

旋转方向的操作，多用于揉、运、摩等手法。关于推拿的左右旋转补泻记载不一。有些穴位旋转补泻的效果不甚明显，但是在腹部，如摩腹、揉中脘、揉神阙等手法，旋转补泻的效果就很明显。在临床操作中，一般认为顺时针方向（向右）旋转为泻法，逆时针方向（向左）旋转为补法。

小儿推拿常用介质

推拿时，在手上蘸些油、粉末或水，在作用于小儿体表穴位时，可以滑润皮肤、增强疗效。这种液体或粉末被称为推拿介质。

滑石粉：即医用滑石粉。有润滑作用——减少摩擦，保护小儿皮肤。一年四季，各种病症均可使用，是临床上最常用的一种介质。

爽身粉：有润滑皮肤、吸水的作用，质量较好的爽身粉可替代滑石粉应用。

薄荷水：取5%薄荷脑5克，加入100毫升75%酒精内配制而成；或取少量薄荷叶，用水浸泡后去渣取汁应用。薄荷水有润滑皮肤、辛凉解表、清暑退热的作用，多用于外感风热，小儿暑热所致的发热、咳嗽等症。

葱、姜水：把葱或生姜捣烂如泥状，放于器皿中，蘸其汁使用；亦可将葱或生姜切片倒入95%酒精，浸出葱、姜汁即可使用。葱、姜汁不仅可润滑皮肤，还有辛温发散的作用，有助于驱散外邪，多用于冬、春季节的风寒表证。

冬青膏：由冬青油、薄荷脑、凡士林和少许麝香配制而成。具有温经散寒和润滑的作用，常用于小儿虚寒性腹泻。

凉水：即凉白开。有清凉退热、润滑皮肤的作用，一般用于小儿外感发热。

香油：即食用香油。在做刮法时，用器具的光滑边缘蘸油，有润滑作用，常用于治疗痧气。

鸡蛋清：将鸡蛋凿一小洞，取其蛋清使用。也可把鸡蛋清与白面和成面团，按摩者手捏面团，在小儿的胸、腹、背部做搓摩滚动。鸡蛋清有润滑皮肤、清热润肺、祛积消食的作用。

小儿推拿的常用手法

小儿经络按摩的手法有十几种，这里介绍几种经常用的，以便读者掌握和应用。

◆推法

用拇指或食指、中指的指腹，在穴位上做单方向的直线推动或环形推动，称为推法。推法分为直推法、旋推法、分推法、合推法四种，其中以直推法应用最多。

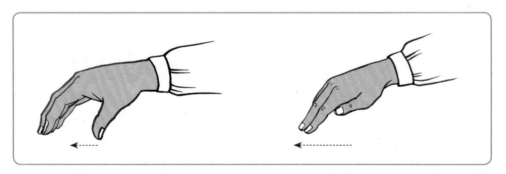

直推法

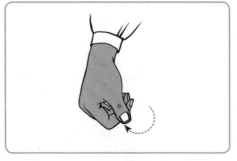

旋推法

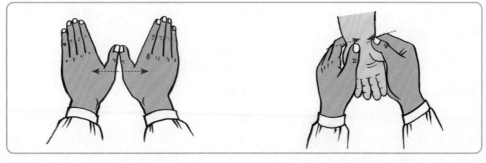

分推法　　　　　　　　　　　　　　　合推法

应用：推法是小儿推拿常用手法之一。直推法常用于头面、上肢、胸腹、腰背和下肢等部位，如推攒竹、推三关、推膻中、推脊、推箕门等，有向上（向心）为"补"、向下（离心）为"清"之说。旋推法主要用于手指的五经穴，如旋推脾经、肺经、肾经等，旋推为补。分推法适用于头面、胸腹、腕掌部和肩胛部，如分推坎宫、分手阴阳、分推膻中、分推肩胛骨、分腹阴阳等，能分利气血。合推法仅用于手腕大横纹，合手阴阳能行痰散结。

◆按法

用手指或掌按压体表，逐渐向下用力，按而留之，称为按法。

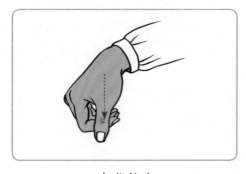　　　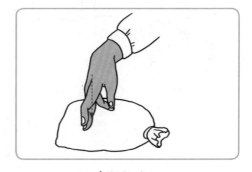

拇指按法　　　　　　　　　　　　　　中指按法

应用：按法刺激性强，指按法多用于点状具有止痛、开窍、止抽搐等作用的穴位。如按环跳、按牙关、按百虫窝。掌按法多用于面状穴位。按法常与揉法配合使用，形成复合手法，缓解刺激，提高疗效，使用范围较广泛。

◆揉法

用手掌大鱼际或掌根、掌心、手指螺纹面着力，吸定于一定部位或穴位上，做顺时针或逆时针方向轻柔和缓的回旋揉动，称为揉法。

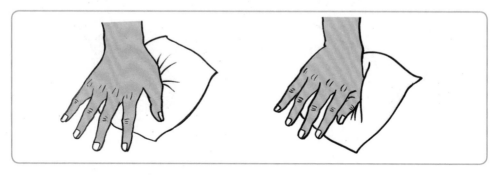

大鱼际揉法

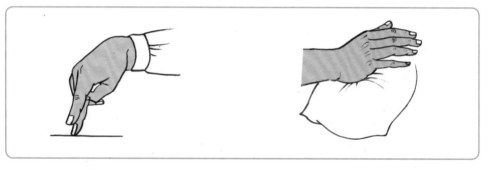

中指揉法　　　　　　　　　　　掌根揉法

应用：揉法刺激量小，作用温和，适用于全身各部位。揉法常与按法、掐法等配合使用，如掐揉二扇门、掐揉小天心等。揉法还常在掐法后使用，即掐后继揉，如掐揉四横纹、掐揉五指节，缓解强刺激手法的不适感。

◆摩法

用手指或手掌，在体表做顺时针或逆时针方向环形按摩，称为摩法。

应用：摩法是小儿按摩常用手法之一，主要用于胸、腹、胁肋部的

面状穴，以腹部应用为多。用于治疗消化不良、便秘、腹泻、疳积等疾病。具有和中理气、消食导滞、调理脾胃、调节肠道功能的作用。

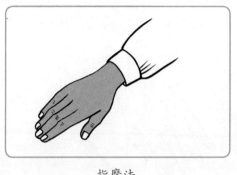
指摩法

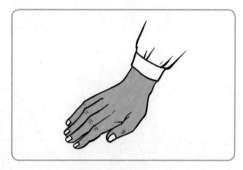
掌摩法

◆掐法

用拇指指甲重刺穴位称掐法。

应用：掐法是强刺激手法之一，适用于头面、手足部穴位，具有定惊醒神、通关开窍的作用。此法以指代针，常用于急症，如急惊风，掐人中、掐十宣、掐老龙，醒神开窍；小儿惊惕不安，掐五指节、掐小天心，以镇惊安神等。

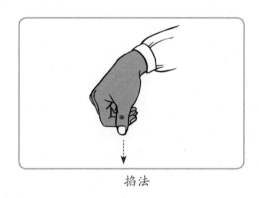
掐法

◆捣法

用中指指端或食指、中指屈曲的指节击打体表一定部位，称为捣法。

应用：捣法相当于指击法，但力量较轻。此法适用于手掌小天心和面部承浆，如捣小天心具有安神定志作用，治疗小儿惊啼。

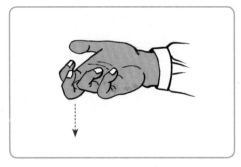

捣法

◆ 运法

用拇指或食指、中指螺纹面在相应穴位上由此至彼，做弧形或环形推动，称运法。

应用：运法是小儿推拿手法中刺激最轻的一种，较旋推法作用面积大。具有理气和血、舒筋活络的作用。运法多用于手掌特定穴，如运水入土、运土入水、运八卦、运板门等。

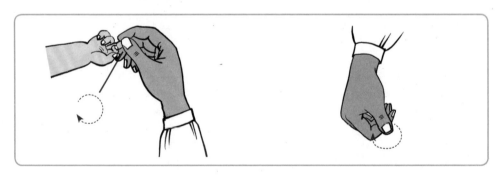

拇指运法

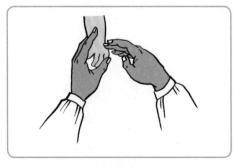

中指运法

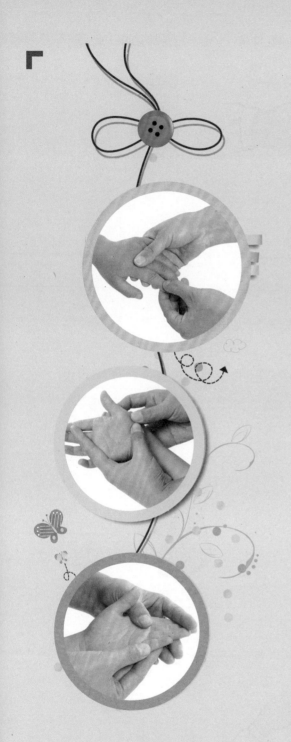

02

小手上的

20个特效穴位

脾经 健脾胃，补气血

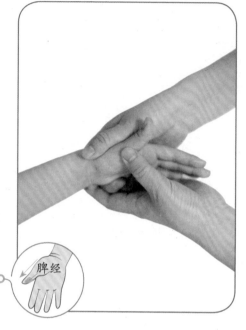

【常用指数】★★★★

【准确定位】拇指桡侧缘或拇指末节螺纹面。

【按摩手法】将小儿拇指伸直，循拇指桡侧边缘由指尖向指根方向直推，或者旋推拇指末节螺纹面，称为补脾经；将小儿拇指伸直，循拇指桡侧缘自指根向指尖方向直推为清，称为清脾经。补脾经和清脾经，统称为推脾经。推100~500次。

【功效作用】补脾经能健脾胃，补气血；清脾经能清热利湿，化痰止呕。

胃经 升食欲，促消化

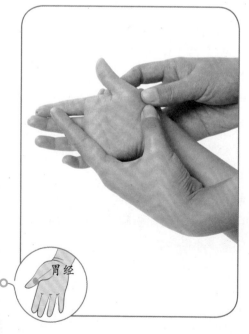

【常用指数】★★★★

【准确定位】拇指掌面近掌端第一节。

【按摩手法】一手托住小儿手，用另一手拇指的指腹或食指和中指的指腹从小儿拇指掌根推至拇指指根，称为清胃经；用拇指螺纹面，旋推小儿拇指掌面近掌端第一节，称为补胃经。清胃经和补胃经，称为推胃经。推100~500次。

【功效作用】补胃经能健脾胃，助运化；清胃经具有清中焦湿热、和胃降逆、泻胃火、除烦止渴的作用。

肝经　驱毒，清热

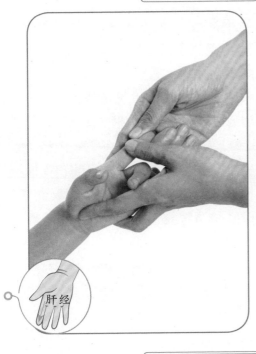

【常用指数】★★★

【准确定位】食指掌面。

【按摩手法】一手托住小儿手，用另一手拇指螺纹面旋推小儿食指螺纹面，称为补肝经；由指根推向指尖，称为清肝经。补肝经和清肝经，统称为推肝经。推100～500次。

【功效作用】清肝经能平肝泻火，息风镇惊，解郁除烦。常用于惊风、抽搐、烦躁不安、五心烦热等症。

心经　清热，退心火

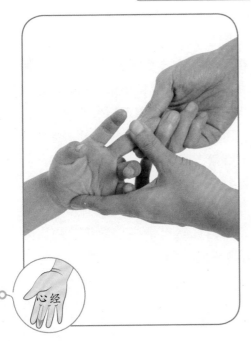

【常用指数】★★★

【准确定位】中指掌面。

【按摩手法】一手托住小儿手，用另一手拇指螺纹面旋推小儿中指螺纹面，称为补心经；从指根推至指尖，称为清心经。补心经和清心经，统称为推心经。推100～500次。

【功效作用】清心经能清热，退心火。常用于心火旺盛而引起的高热神昏、面赤口疮、小便短赤等症。

肺经　宣肺，清热，止咳

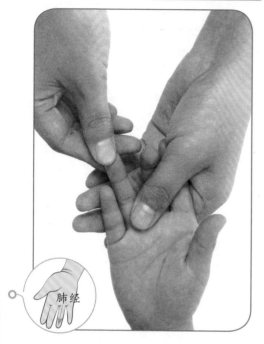

肺经

【常用指数】★★★★

【准确定位】无名指掌面。

【按摩手法】一手托住小儿手，用另一手拇指螺纹面旋推小儿无名指螺纹面，称为补肺经；从指根直推至指尖，称为清肺经。补肺经和清肺经，统称为推肺经。推100～500次。

【功效作用】补肺经能补益肺气，清肺经可宣肺清热。

肾经　补肾，益脑，治腹泻

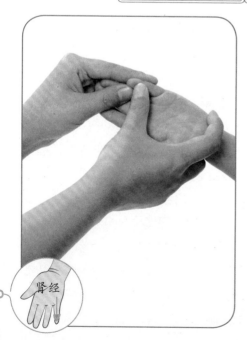

肾经

【常用指数】★★★

【准确定位】小指掌面。

【按摩手法】一手托住小儿手，再用另一手拇指指腹由小儿小指指根向指尖方向直推，或者旋推小指末节螺纹面，称为补肾经；由指尖向指根方向直推，称为清肾经。补肾经和清肾经，统称为推肾经。推100～500次。

【功效作用】补肾经能补肾益脑，温养下元；清肾经能清利下焦湿热。

大肠经 通便，止泻

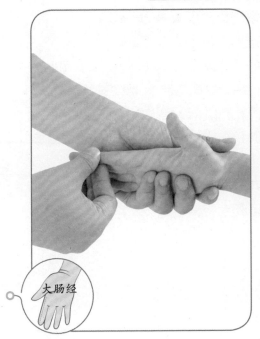

大肠经

【常用指数】★★★★

【准确定位】食指桡侧缘，自食指尖至虎口成一直线。

【按摩手法】一手托住小儿手，使之暴露桡侧缘，用另一手拇指指腹从小儿食指指尖直推向虎口为补，称为补大肠经；反之为清，称为清大肠经。补大肠经和清大肠经，统称为推大肠经。推100~300次。

【功效作用】补大肠经能涩肠固脱，温中止泻；清大肠经能清利肠腑，除湿热，导积滞。

四横纹 治积食，助消化

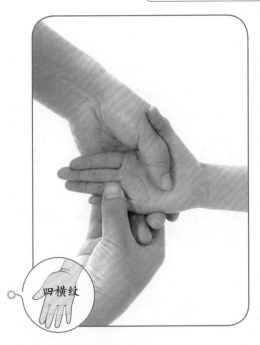

四横纹

【常用指数】★★★★

【准确定位】在掌面食指、中指、无名指、小指第一指间关节横纹处。

【按摩手法】一手托住小儿手，使掌心向上，用另一手拇指从小儿食指依次掐揉至小指横纹，称为掐揉四横纹，掐揉3~5次；四指并拢，从食指横纹推向小指横纹处，来回推，称为推四横纹，推100~300次。四横纹有掐法、揉法、推法3种操作。

【功效作用】掐揉四横纹是治疗小儿疳积的要穴，能退热除烦，散瘀结；推四横纹能调中行气，和气血，消胀满。

板门（大鱼际）　胃口好，吃饭香

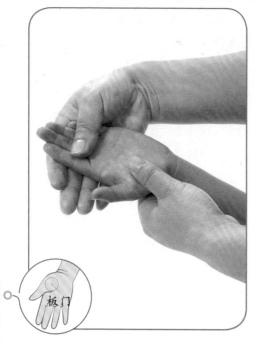

板门

【常用指数】★★★★

【准确定位】手掌大鱼际平面。

【按摩手法】一手托住小儿手，用另一手拇指端揉小儿大鱼际，称为揉板门或运板门，揉50～100次；用推法时，自拇指根推向腕横纹，称为板门推向横纹，反之称为横纹推向板门，推100～300次。板门穴有揉法、运法、推法3种操作。

【功效作用】揉板门能健脾和胃，消食化滞，运达上下之气。板门推向横纹，健脾止泻；横纹推向板门，降逆止呕。

内劳宫　清热除烦，退心火

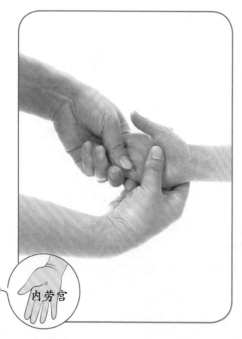

内劳宫

【常用指数】★★★★

【准确定位】手掌心中，屈指时中指、无名指指端之间中点。

【按摩手法】一手托住小儿手，用另一手拇指或中指端揉小儿掌心，称为揉内劳宫，揉100～300次；用拇指螺纹面或中指端运内劳宫，称为运内劳宫，运10～30次。内劳宫有揉法和运法2种操作。

【功效作用】揉内劳宫能清热除烦，运内劳宫具有清心、肾两经虚热作用。

内八卦　除百病

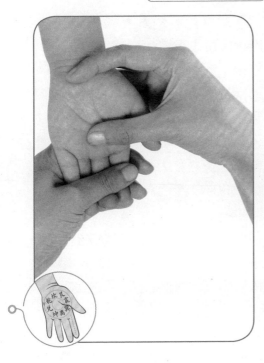

【常用指数】★★★★★

【准确定位】手掌面，以掌心为圆心，从圆心至中指根横纹约2/3处为半径做圆周。八卦穴在此圆周上，即乾、坎、艮、震、巽、离、坤、兑8个方位。

【按摩手法】一手持小儿四指，使其掌心向上，用另一手食指、中指夹住小儿腕关节，以拇指螺纹面用运法。自乾宫起，顺时针向坎宫施运，至兑宫止，周而复始，称为运八卦，运100～500次；自艮宫起，逆时针向坎宫施运，至震宫止，周而复始，称为逆运八卦，运100～500次。

【功效作用】运八卦能宽胸利膈，理气化痰，行滞消食；逆运八卦能降气平喘。

小天心　清心安神

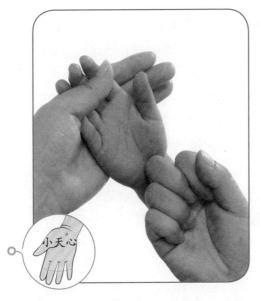

【常用指数】★★★★★

【准确定位】大、小鱼际交接凹陷中。

【按摩手法】一手持小儿四指，使掌心向上，用另一手中指端揉，称为揉小天心，揉100～300次；用拇指指甲掐，称为掐小天心，掐3～5次；用中指尖或屈曲的指间关节捣，称为捣小天心，捣10～30次。小天心有揉法、掐法、捣法3种操作。

【功效作用】掐揉小天心具有清热、镇惊、利尿、明目的作用；掐捣小天心能镇静安神。

二扇门　快速清火退热

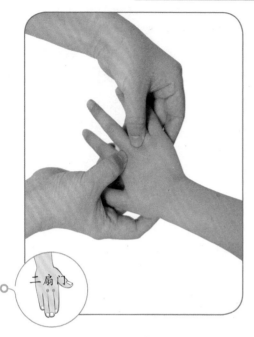

二扇门

【常用指数】★★★★★

【准确定位】掌背处中指根本节两侧凹陷处。

【按摩手法】用两手食指、中指夹住小儿手掌，使其手心向下，用两拇指指甲掐之，称为掐二扇门，掐3~5次；用两拇指偏峰按揉之，或一手握小儿手腕，用另一手食指、中指按揉之，称为揉二扇门，揉300~500次。

【功效作用】掐、揉二扇门处能发汗透表，退热平喘，是发汗效穴。揉时要稍用力，速度宜快，多用于风寒外感。

二人上马　滋阴补肾，顺气散结

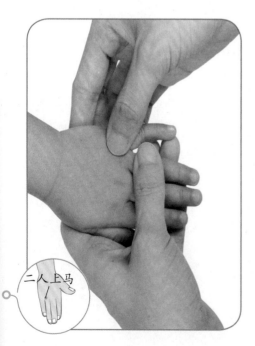

二人上马

【常用指数】★★★★★

【准确定位】手背无名指及小指掌指关节后陷中。

【按摩手法】一手握小儿四指，使掌心向下，用另一手拇指掐之，称为掐二人上马，掐3~5次；或用拇指、中指相对用力揉之，称为揉二人上马，揉300~500次。

【功效作用】揉二人上马能滋阴补肾，顺气散结，利水通淋，为补肾滋阴的要法。

外劳宫　祛体寒，治感冒

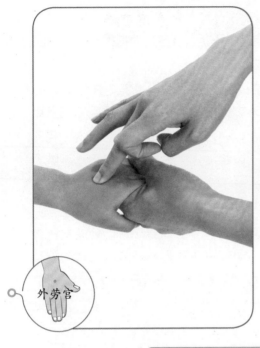

外劳宫

【常用指数】★ ★ ★ ★

【准确定位】掌背正中第三、第四掌骨中间凹陷处，与内劳宫相对。

【按摩手法】一手握小儿四指，用另一手拇指或中指端揉之，称为揉外劳宫，揉100~300次；用拇指指甲掐之，称为掐外劳宫，掐3~5次。

【功效作用】揉外劳宫具有温阳散寒、升阳举陷作用，兼能发汗解表。本法性温，用于寒证。

外八卦　治腹胀，除便秘

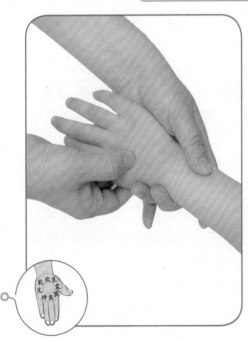

【常用指数】★ ★ ★

【准确定位】手背外劳宫周围，与内八卦相对处。

【按摩手法】一手托住小儿手，使掌背向上，用另一手拇指，做顺时针方向掐运，称为运外八卦，运100~300次。

【功效作用】运外八卦能宽胸理气，通滞散结，可治疗胸闷、腹胀、便结等症，常与运八卦、推揉膻中、摩腹等合用。

一窝风　发散风寒，治腹痛

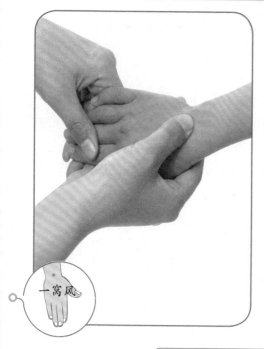

一窝风

【常用指数】★ ★ ★ ★

【准确定位】手背腕横纹正中凹陷处。

【按摩手法】一手持小儿手掌，使掌背向上，用另一手中指或拇指揉之，称为揉一窝风，揉100～300次。

【功效作用】揉一窝风能温中行气，止痹痛，利关节，用于受寒、食积等原因引起的腹痛等症。

天河水　退热，去火

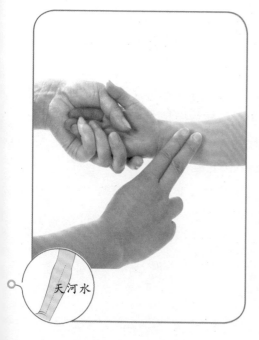

天河水

【常用指数】★ ★ ★ ★ ★

【准确定位】前臂内侧正中，总筋至洪池（曲泽）成一直线。

【按摩手法】一手握小儿手，使其掌心向上，用另一手食指、中指指面从小儿腕横纹推向肘横纹，称为推天河水或清天河水，推100～500次；用食指、中指蘸水自小儿总筋处，一起一落弹打如弹琴状，直至洪池，同时用口吹气随之，称为弹打天河水或打马过天河，5～6下一回，拍打100～300回。

【功效作用】清天河水能清热解表，泻火除烦。本法性微凉，清热较平和，用于治疗热性病症。

三关 发汗解表，补气血

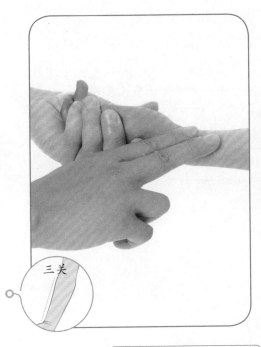

三关

【常用指数】★★★★★

【准确定位】前臂桡侧，阳池至曲池成一直线。

【按摩手法】一手握小儿手，用另一手拇指桡侧面或食指、中指指面从小儿手腕推向肘部，称为推三关；屈小儿拇指，自拇指外侧推向肘，称为大推三关。推100～300次。

【功效作用】推三关能补气行气，温阳散寒，发汗解表。本法性温热，主治虚寒病症，对非虚寒病症者宜慎用。

六腑 清热解毒，息风定惊

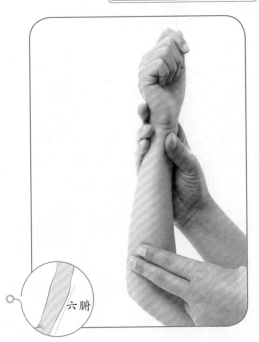

六腑

【常用指数】★★★★★

【准确定位】前臂尺侧，肘至阴池成一直线。

【按摩手法】一手握住小儿手腕，用另一手拇指或食指和中指的指面自小儿肘部尺侧端，推至腕掌侧横纹尺侧端，称为退六腑。推100～500次。

【功效作用】退六腑能清热，解毒，凉血。本法性寒凉，用于实热病症。

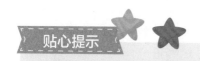

贴心提示

1. 以五脏命名的穴位脾经、肝经、心经、肺经、肾经，可治疗本脏的病症，用补法能补其不足，用清法能泻其有余。其中肝经、心经两穴宜清不宜补，若补时，须补后加清；脾经、肾经两穴用补法为多，清法宜少用；唯肺经有补有泻。五穴组合又称五经穴，与相关的脏腑经穴相配，治疗相关脏腑病症。

2. 以六腑命名的穴位，胃经、大肠经和小肠经，主要用于治疗本腑的病症，用补法能补其不足，用清法能泻其有余，但其中胃经、小肠经多用清法。

3. 掐揉二扇门、清天河水、揉外劳宫、掐揉一窝风、推三关，五法均能解肌发表，治疗外感病，但掐揉二扇门发汗作用较强，宜用于邪实体壮者。清天河水主要用于外感风热，后三法兼能温阳散寒，主要用于外感风寒。而推三关又能补益气血，揉外劳宫兼散脏腑积寒和升阳举陷，掐揉一窝风也可治腹痛。

4. 清天河水、退六腑、掐揉小天心、揉内劳宫、运内劳宫、揉二人上马，这几法均能清热。而清天河水主要清卫分、气分之热；退六腑主要清营分、血分之热；运内劳宫、揉二人上马清虚烦内热；揉内劳宫、掐揉小天心主要清心经之热，而后者兼有利尿、镇惊的作用，用于心经有热，或移热于小肠、惊惕不安、小便短赤者。分阴阳能调和气血，主要用于寒热往来，气血不和。

5. 推板门、揉板门、揉端正、运八卦、运外八卦，这几法均能健脾和中，助运消滞。揉板门主要能消食化滞；板门推向横纹、揉左端正主治腹泻；横纹推向板门、揉右端正主治呕吐；运八卦、运外八卦兼能宽胸理气，而前者又能止咳化痰。

6. 掐揉四横纹、揉掌小横纹、推小横纹、揉肾纹、掐揉总筋，这几法均能清热散结，而掐揉四横纹主和气血，消食积，是治疗疳积的要穴；揉掌小横纹主清心、肺之热结，治疗肺部湿性啰音；推小横纹主清脾、胃热结，调中消胀，治疗肺部干性啰音；揉肾纹清心、肝之热结，祛风明目；揉总筋兼通调周身气机，清心止痉，治口舌生疮。

7. 推三关与退六腑是大凉大热之法，可单用，亦可合用。气虚体弱，畏寒怕冷，可单用推三关；高热烦渴、发斑等可单用退六腑；合用能平衡阴阳，防止大凉大热，伤及正气。寒热夹杂，以热为主，退六腑3次，推三关1次，即3：1推之，通常称为退三推一法；若以寒为重，退六腑1次，则推三关3次，即1：3，称为推三退一法。

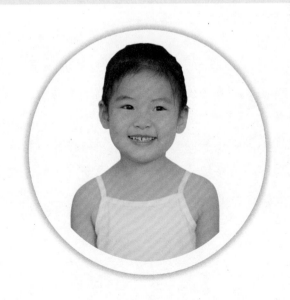

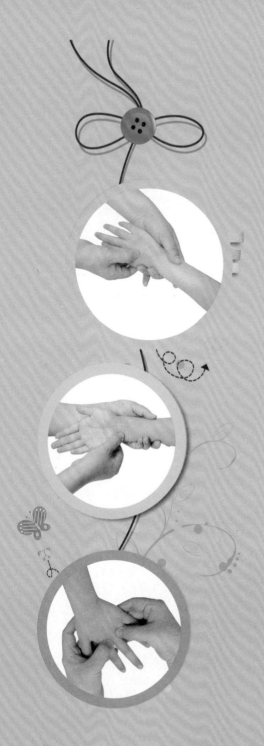

推拿治疗
15种小儿常见病

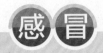

感冒

　　感冒是困扰小儿的常见病之一，四季均有发生，尤以秋、冬季节多见。中医认为，感冒多由风寒或风热从口鼻肌表侵犯肺系所致，常以发热、恶寒、鼻塞流涕、咳嗽为特征，在气候突变、寒温失常、坐卧当风、养护不当时易诱发感冒。治疗原则以解表、散寒、清热为主。

手部穴位精解

清肝经

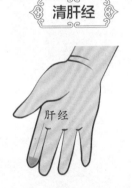

肝经

【准确定位】食指掌面。

【按摩手法】一手托住小儿手，使掌心向上，用另一手拇指指腹从小儿食指指根直推至指尖。

【功效作用】清热，排毒。

清肺经

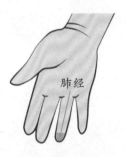

肺经

【准确定位】无名指掌面。

【按摩手法】一手托住小儿手，使掌心向上，用另一手拇指指腹从小儿无名指指根直推至指尖。

【功效作用】宣肺清热，疏风解表，化痰止咳。

清天河水

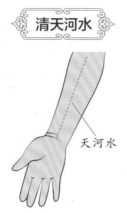

天河水

【准确定位】前臂内侧正中，总筋至洪池成一直线。

【按摩手法】一手握住小儿手，使掌心向上，用另一手食指和中指指腹自小儿腕横纹推向肘横纹。

【功效作用】清心除烦，镇惊安神，退热发表。

退六腑

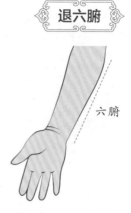

六腑

【准确定位】前臂尺侧，肘至阴池成一直线。

【按摩手法】一手握住小儿手腕，用另一手食指、中指指腹自小儿肘横纹尺侧端推至腕掌侧横纹尺侧端。

【功效作用】清热解毒，消肿止痛。

掐五指节

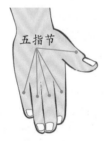

五指节

【准确定位】五指背侧第一指骨间关节。

【按摩手法】一手托住小儿手，使其手背向上，用另一手拇指指甲依次从小儿拇指掐至小指。

【功效作用】安神镇惊，祛风痰，通关窍。

清胃经

胃经

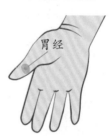

【准确定位】拇指的掌面近掌端第一节。

【按摩手法】一手托住小儿手，使掌心向上，用另一手拇指指腹从小儿拇指掌根推至拇指指根。

【功效作用】清胃热，降胃气。

运八卦

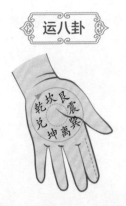

【准确定位】掌中，围绕掌心内劳宫一周，按乾、坎、艮、震、巽、离、坤、兑八卦分布。

【按摩手法】一手托住小儿手，使掌心向上，用另一手拇指指腹自小儿乾宫起顺时针做运法。

【功效作用】宽胸利膈，理气化痰，行滞消食。

清大肠经

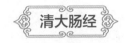

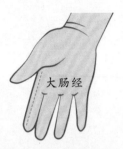

【准确定位】食指桡侧缘，自食指尖到虎口成一直线。

【按摩手法】一手托住小儿手，露出食指桡侧缘，用另一手拇指指腹由小儿虎口直推至指尖。

【功效作用】清利大肠，除湿热。

捣小天心

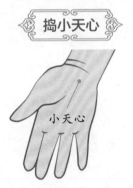

【准确定位】在大、小鱼际交界处凹陷中，在劳宫与腕掌侧横纹之间。

【按摩手法】一手托住小儿手，使掌心向上，用另一手屈曲中指以第一指间关节捣小儿小天心。

【功效作用】镇静安神，醒脑开窍，清热除烦。

揉阳池

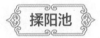

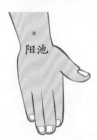

【准确定位】手背一窝风上3寸凹陷处。

【按摩手法】一手握小儿手腕，使掌背向上，用另一手拇指和中指指端相对用力揉小儿本穴。

【功效作用】降逆，清脑，祛风止痛。

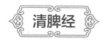

清脾经

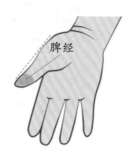

脾经

【准确定位】拇指桡侧缘或拇指末节螺纹面。

【按摩手法】一手持小儿手掌，使掌心向上，将小儿拇指伸直，沿拇指桡侧缘，自指根直推至指尖。

【功效作用】健脾胃，清热利湿。

一般感冒

【症状表现】恶寒发热，头痛，四肢关节痛，鼻塞流涕，咳嗽喷嚏等。

【治疗原则】解表，散寒，清热。

【按摩频率】每天按摩2次，按摩后以微汗出、自觉舒适为宜，切勿发汗太过。

发热低于 39℃

1. 清肺经5分钟：

用拇指指腹从无名指掌面指根直推至指尖。

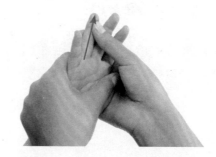

2. 清天河水5分钟：

用食指和中指指腹自掌侧腕横纹推向肘横纹。

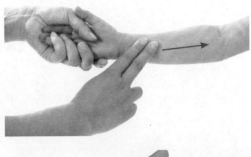

3. 掐五指节1分钟：

用拇指指甲自拇指至小指依次掐五指背侧第一指骨间关节。

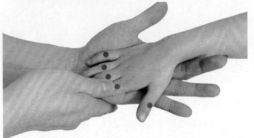

高热时（39～40℃）

1. 掐五指节3分钟：

用拇指指甲自拇指至小指依次掐五指背侧第一指骨间关节。

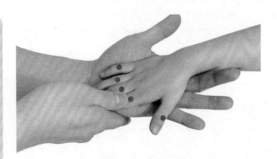

2. 退六腑5分钟：

用食指、中指指腹自肘部尺侧推向手腕尺侧。

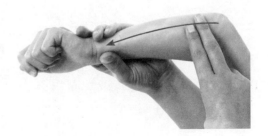

3. 感冒鼻塞重，加揉阳池5分钟：

用拇指和中指指端相对用力揉手背一窝风上3寸凹陷处。

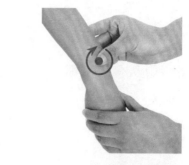

4. 感冒伴呕吐，加清胃经5分钟：

用拇指指腹自拇指掌根推至拇指指根。

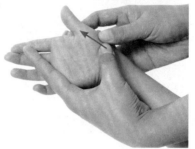

5. 感冒咳嗽重，加运八卦5分钟：

用拇指指腹自乾宫起顺时针做运法。

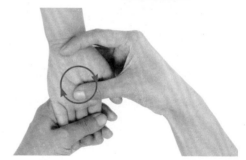

感冒夹痰

【症状表现】兼见咳喘，舌苔微黄腻或黏，脉浮滑数。

【治疗原则】解表，祛风热，宽胸，理气，化痰。

【按摩频率】每天按摩2次，按摩后以微汗出、自觉舒适为宜，切勿发汗太过。

1. 清肝经5分钟：

用拇指指腹从食指掌面指根直推至指尖。

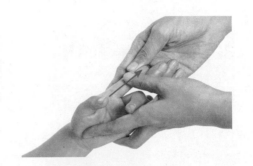

2. 运八卦5分钟：

用拇指指腹自乾宫起顺时针做运法。

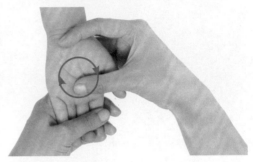

3. 清天河水5分钟：

用食指和中指指腹自掌侧腕横纹推向肘横纹。

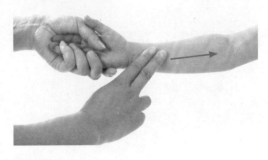

4. 痰盛，加清补脾经5分钟：

用拇指指腹循拇指桡侧缘，从指根到指尖来回推。

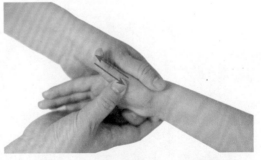

5. 高热，加退六腑5分钟：

用食指、中指指腹自肘部尺侧推向手腕尺侧。

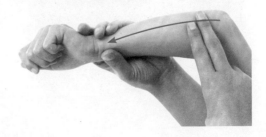

感冒夹滞

【症状表现】纳呆吐泻，腹胀肠鸣，或见高热，舌苔黄厚，脉滑实。

【治疗原则】解表，祛风热，理气化积。

【按摩频率】每天按摩2次，按摩后以微汗出、自觉舒适为宜，切勿发汗太过。

1. 清天河水5分钟：

用食指和中指指腹自掌侧腕横纹推向肘横纹。

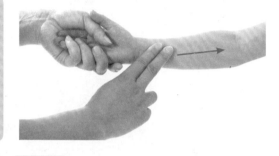

2. 清脾经5分钟：

用拇指指腹循拇指桡侧缘，从指根推向指尖。

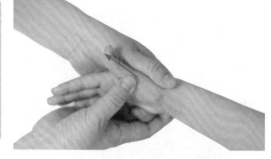

3. 清胃经5分钟：

用拇指指腹自拇指掌根推至拇指指根。

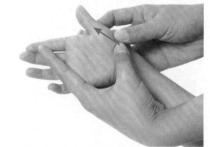

4. 清大肠经5分钟：

用拇指指腹推食指桡侧，由虎口直推至食指指尖。

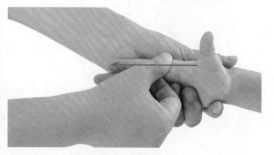

感冒夹惊

【症状表现】烦躁惊厥，高热，甚或角弓反张，苔黄偏干，脉弦数。

【治疗原则】解表，祛风热，息肝风，安神镇惊。

【按摩频率】每天按摩2次，按摩后以微汗出、自觉舒适为宜，切勿发汗太过。

1. 清肝经20分钟：

用拇指指腹从食指掌面指根直推至指尖。

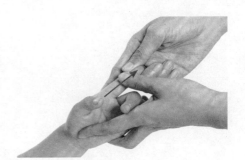

2. 清天河水20分钟：

用食指和中指指腹自掌侧腕横纹推向肘横纹。

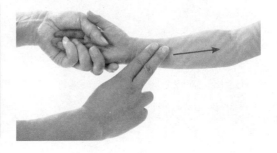

3. 高热，加退六腑5分钟：

用食指、中指指腹自肘部尺侧推向手腕尺侧。

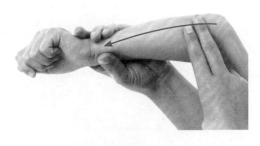

4. 如见角弓反张、目上翻、惊厥等症状，加捣小天心1~2分钟：

屈曲中指以第一指间关节捣小天心。

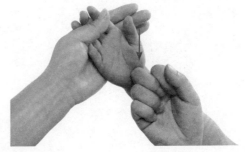

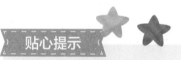

食疗小偏方

姜糖饮：

生姜片15克，葱白适量，红糖20克。葱白切段，与生姜一起，加水100毫升煮沸3~5分钟，加入红糖即可。趁热一次性服下，盖被取微汗。可治疗感冒头痛、身痛无汗。

葱白粥：

粳米50克，葱白、白糖各适量。粳米煮熟后，把切成段的葱白2~3段及白糖放入即可。每日1次，热服，取微汗。可解表散寒，适用于风寒感冒。

贴心提示

孩子感冒发热多由风寒引起，可给孩子吃热的稀粥，避风，穿暖衣或盖被捂至微出汗。感冒自然病程约1周，如果感冒症状持续超过1周，可能并发其他疾病，应去医院就诊。

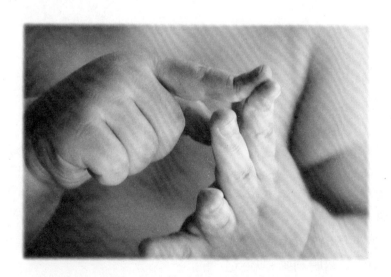

支气管炎

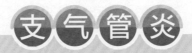

　　小儿支气管炎发病时，会出现咳嗽、发热、胸痛、咳痰、呕吐、呼吸困难等症状，属于中医风温病的范畴。中医认为，本病主要是肺部受风寒所致。对于急性支气管炎，治疗原则以解表清肺和止咳化痰为主；慢性支气管炎的治疗原则以健脾益气和止咳平喘为主。

手部穴位精解

运八卦

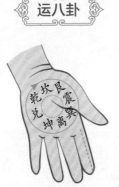

【准确定位】掌中，围绕掌心内劳宫一周，按乾、坎、艮、震、巽、离、坤、兑八卦分布。

【按摩手法】一手托住小儿手，使掌心向上，用另一手拇指指腹自小儿乾宫起顺时针做运法。

【功效作用】宽胸利膈，理气化痰，行滞消食。

清肝经

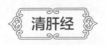
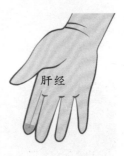

【准确定位】食指掌面。

【按摩手法】一手托住小儿手，使掌心向上，用另一手拇指指腹从小儿食指指根直推至指尖。

【功效作用】清热，排毒。

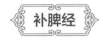

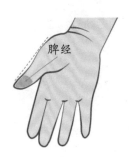

【准确定位】拇指桡侧缘或拇指末节螺纹面。

【按摩手法】一手持小儿小指，用另一手拇指指腹旋推小儿拇指末节螺纹面。

【功效作用】健脾胃，补气血。

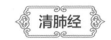

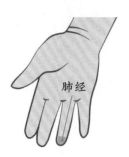

【准确定位】无名指掌面。

【按摩手法】一手托住小儿手，使掌心向上，用另一手拇指指腹从小儿无名指指根直推至指尖。

【功效作用】宣肺清热，疏风解表，化痰止咳。

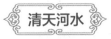

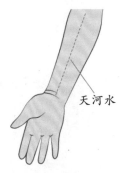

【准确定位】前臂内侧正中，总筋至洪池成一直线。

【按摩手法】一手握住小儿手，使掌心向上，用另一手食指和中指指腹自小儿腕横纹推向肘横纹。

【功效作用】清心除烦，镇惊安神，退热发表。

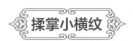

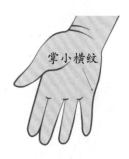

【准确定位】掌面小指根下，尺侧掌纹头。

【按摩手法】一手持小儿手，用另一手拇指或中指端按揉小儿本穴。

【功效作用】清热散结，宽胸宣肺，化痰止咳。

揉二人上马

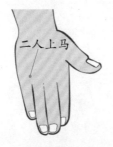

二人上马

【准确定位】手背无名指与小指掌指关节后凹陷中。

【按摩手法】用双手拇指、中指相对按揉小儿本穴。

【功效作用】引火归原，补肾利水，顺气散结。

推四横纹

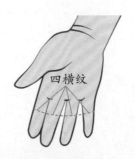

四横纹

【准确定位】掌面食指、中指、无名指、小指第一指间关节横纹处。

【按摩手法】一手持小儿手，使掌心向上，用另一手拇指指腹从小儿食指横纹推向小指横纹处，来回推。

【功效作用】调中行气，和气血，消胀满。

退六腑

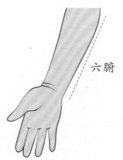

六腑

【准确定位】前臂尺侧，肘至阴池成一直线。

【按摩手法】一手握住小儿手腕，用另一手食指、中指指腹自小儿肘横纹尺侧端推至腕掌侧横纹尺侧端。

【功效作用】清热解毒，消肿止痛。

逆运八卦

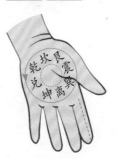

乾 坎 艮 震 巽 离 坤 兑

【准确定位】掌中，围绕掌心内劳宫一周，按乾、坎、艮、震、巽、离、坤、兑八卦分布。

【按摩手法】一手托住小儿手，使掌心向上，用另一手拇指指腹自小儿艮宫起逆时针做运法。

【功效作用】降气平喘。

急性支气管炎

【症状表现】初起有感冒症状，继则咳嗽加重，可有发热、胸闷、气促、食欲缺乏等症状。初为干咳，以后痰渐多。

【治疗原则】解表清肺，止咳化痰。

【按摩频率】每天按摩2次，不拘疗程，直至痊愈。

1. 运八卦5分钟：

用拇指指腹自乾宫起顺时针做运法。

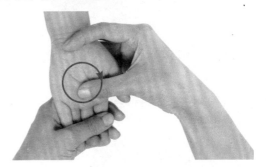

2. 清肝经5分钟：

用拇指指腹从食指掌面指根直推至指尖。

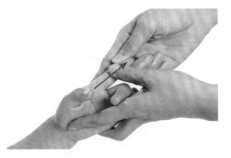

3. 清肺经5分钟：

用拇指指腹从无名指掌面指根直推至指尖。

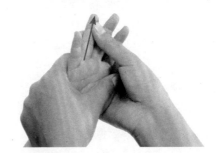

4. 清天河水5分钟：

用食指和中指指腹自腕掌侧横纹推至肘横纹。

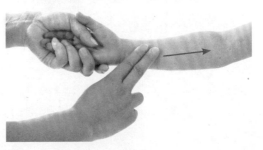

5. 发热38.5℃以上，加退六腑5分钟：

用食指、中指指腹自肘部尺侧推向手腕尺侧。

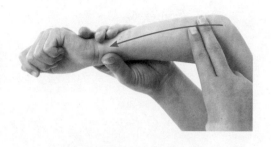

6. 喘重痰多，加揉掌小横纹5分钟：

用拇指指腹揉掌面小指根下尺侧掌纹头。

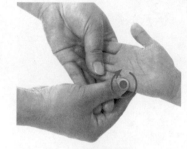

7. 唯独喘重，少痰或无痰，揉掌小横纹改用推四横纹5分钟：

用拇指指腹从食指横纹推向小指横纹，来回推。

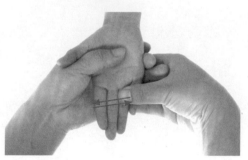

慢性支气管炎

【症状表现】急性支气管炎如反复发作，可发展为慢性支气管炎。轻者仅早晚咳嗽，重者可有发热、咳嗽、吐痰明显、活动后喘、呼吸可带哮鸣声、日渐消瘦等表现。

【治疗原则】健脾益气，止咳平喘。

【按摩频率】每天2次，不拘疗程，直至痊愈。

1. 补脾经5分钟：

用拇指指腹旋推拇指末节螺纹面。

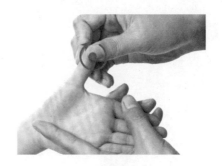

2. 清肺经5分钟：

用拇指指腹从无名指掌面指根直推至指尖。

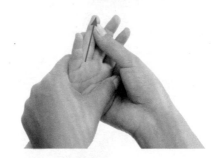

3. 揉二人上马5分钟：

用拇指、中指指腹相对用力揉手背无名指与小指掌指关节后凹陷处。

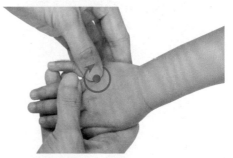

4. 逆运八卦5分钟：

用拇指指腹自艮宫起逆时针做运法。

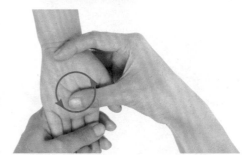

食疗小偏方

沙参百合茶饮：

沙参15克，百合15克，川贝母3克。共研粗末，冲入沸水，加盖焖30分钟。代茶饮用，每日1剂。治燥热型急性支气管炎，症见干咳无痰或痰中带血，鼻燥，咽干，咳甚则胸痛，大便干燥，小便黄少。

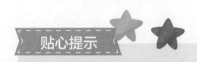

贴心提示

咳嗽可由多种疾病引起，尤其是伴有发热超过3天或咳嗽剧烈的情况下，应及时就诊。孩子咳嗽时，不适合吃川贝炖梨，往往会越吃越严重。川贝母和梨有滋阴润燥和止咳化痰的作用，对老年人长期阴虚咳嗽疗效较好，不适合孩子服用。

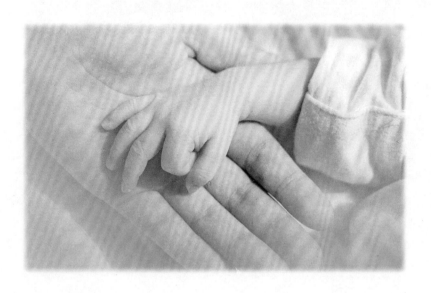

肺炎是小儿常见病，也是严重危及小儿健康甚至生命的疾病。肺炎四季皆可见，尤以冬、春季常见。中医认为，引起小儿肺炎的原因主要是感受风邪、邪气闭肺，邪热炽盛、热邪闭肺。症状表现为不同程度的发热、咳嗽、呼吸急促、呼吸困难和肺部啰音等。治疗原则以清肺化痰为主。但也有些幼儿患上肺炎，症状常不明显，可能仅有轻微咳嗽或完全没有咳嗽，应注意及时治疗。

手部穴位精解

清肝经

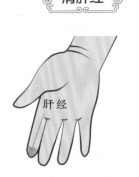

肝经

【准确定位】食指掌面。

【按摩手法】一手托住小儿手，使掌心向上，用另一手拇指指腹从小儿食指指根直推至指尖。

【功效作用】清热，排毒。

清肺经

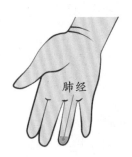

肺经

【准确定位】无名指掌面。

【按摩手法】一手托住小儿手，使掌心向上，用另一手拇指指腹从小儿无名指指根直推至指尖。

【功效作用】宣肺清热，疏风解表，化痰止咳。

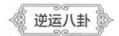

逆运八卦

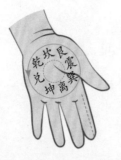

【准确定位】掌中，围绕掌心内劳宫一周，按乾、坎、艮、震、巽、离、坤、兑八卦分布。

【按摩手法】一手托住小儿手，使掌心向上，用另一手拇指指腹自小儿艮宫起逆时针做运法。

【功效作用】降气平喘。

退六腑

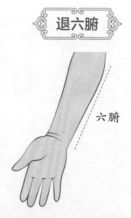

六腑

【准确定位】前臂尺侧，肘至阴池成一直线。

【按摩手法】一手握住小儿手腕，用另一手食指、中指指腹自小儿肘横纹尺侧端推至腕掌侧横纹尺侧端。

【功效作用】清热解毒，消肿止痛。

揉掌小横纹

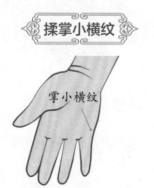

掌小横纹

【准确定位】掌面小指根下，尺侧掌纹头。

【按摩手法】一手持小儿手，用另一手拇指或中指端按揉小儿本穴。

【功效作用】清热散结，宽胸宣肺，化痰止咳。

清心经

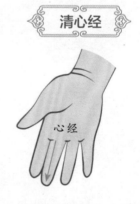

心经

【准确定位】掌面，中指指面。

【按摩手法】一手持小儿手，另一手拇指指腹从小儿中指指根直推至指尖。

【功效作用】清热，退心火。

捣小天心

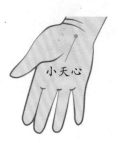

小天心

【准确定位】在大、小鱼际交界处凹陷中，在劳宫与腕掌侧横纹之间。

【按摩手法】一手托住小儿手，使掌心向上，用另一手屈曲中指以第一指间关节捣小儿小天心。

【功效作用】镇静安神，醒脑开窍，清热除烦。

揉阳池

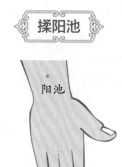

阳池

【准确定位】手背一窝风上3寸凹陷处。

【按摩手法】一手握小儿手腕，使掌背向上，用另一手拇指和中指指端相对用力揉小儿本穴。

【功效作用】降逆，清脑，祛风止痛。

普通肺炎

【症状表现】初起发热、咳嗽、流涕、食欲缺乏、有时呕吐，继则出现呼吸困难。

【治疗原则】清肺化痰。

【按摩频率】每天2次，不拘疗程，直至痊愈。

1. 清肝经5分钟：

用拇指指腹从食指掌面指根直推至指尖。

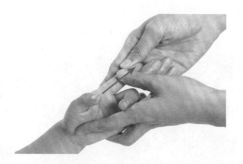

2. 清肺经5分钟：

用拇指指腹从无名指掌面指根直推至指尖。

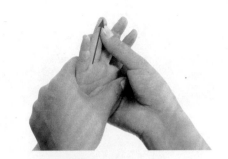

3. 逆运八卦5分钟：

用拇指指腹自艮宫起逆时针做运法。

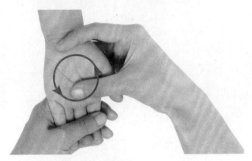

4. 揉掌小横纹5分钟：

用拇指指腹揉掌面小指根下尺侧掌纹头。

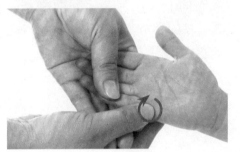

5. 退六腑5分钟：

用食指、中指指腹自肘部尺侧推向手腕尺侧。

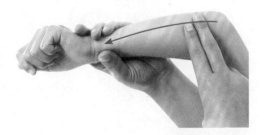

6. 痰盛，加清心经3分钟：

用拇指指腹从中指掌面指根直推至指尖。

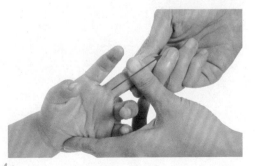

7. 若高热引起惊厥，加捣小天心1～2分钟：

屈曲中指以第一指间关节捣小天心。

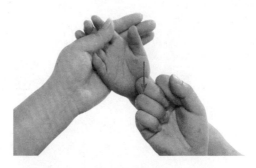

8. 若头痛鼻塞，加揉阳池5分钟：

用拇指和中指指端相对用力揉手背一窝风上3寸凹陷处。

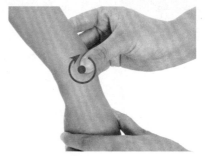

食疗小偏方

银耳莲子鸡汤：

　　银耳15克，莲子60克，鸡汤1500克，白糖适量。将银耳、莲子泡发、蒸熟；鸡汤煮沸后加白糖、银耳、莲子，再次煮沸即成。每日3剂，连服3～5剂。

萝卜牛肺二冬汤：

　　萝卜、牛肺各500克，麦冬30克，天冬20克，甜杏仁15克，生姜及调味品适量。将牛肺、白萝卜洗净、切块，与麦冬、天冬、甜杏仁同放砂锅中，武火煮沸，转文火炖至烂后，加姜等调味服食。每日1剂，连服3～5剂。

贴心提示

　　肺炎通常会引起高热，但年龄较小或体质较弱的小儿常常不发热或仅有低热，但有咳嗽、咳痰等症状，应引起重视，及时就医。

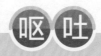

呕吐在婴幼儿时期较为常见，可见于多种病症。如急性胃炎、贲门痉挛、幽门痉挛、幽门梗阻等，呕吐属于主症之一。中医认为，引起呕吐的原因主要是外感邪气（如受凉）、内伤乳食、大惊猝恐以及其他脏腑疾病影响到胃的正常功能，导致胃失和降、胃气上逆，从而引起呕吐。治疗原则以清胃和中和降逆止呕为主。

手部穴位精解

清胃经

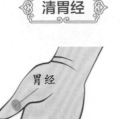

胃经

【准确定位】拇指掌面近掌端第一节。

【按摩手法】一手托住小儿手，使掌心向上，用另一手拇指指腹从小儿拇指掌根推至拇指指根。

【功效作用】清胃热，降胃气。

清肝经

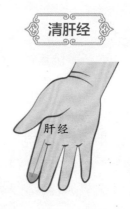

肝经

【准确定位】食指掌面。

【按摩手法】一手托住小儿手，使掌心向上，用另一手拇指指腹从小儿食指指根直推至指尖。

【功效作用】清热，排毒。

清天河水

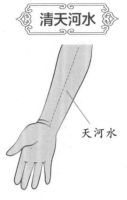

天河水

【准确定位】前臂内侧正中，总筋至洪池成一直线。

【按摩手法】一手握住小儿手，使掌心向上，用另一手食指和中指指腹自小儿腕横纹推向肘横纹。

【功效作用】清心除烦，镇惊安神，退热发表。

运八卦

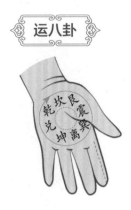

乾坎艮震巽离坤兑

【准确定位】掌中，围绕掌心内劳宫一周，按乾、坎、艮、震、巽、离、坤、兑八卦分布。

【按摩手法】一手托住小儿手，使掌心向上，用另一手拇指指腹自小儿乾宫起顺时针做运法。

【功效作用】宽胸利膈，理气化痰，行滞消食。

清大肠经

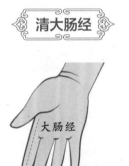

大肠经

【准确定位】食指桡侧缘，自食指尖到虎口成一直线。

【按摩手法】一手托住小儿手，露出食指桡侧缘，用另一手拇指指腹由小儿虎口直推至指尖。

【功效作用】清利大肠，除湿热。

揉板门

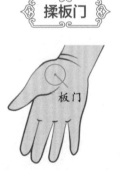

板门

【准确定位】手掌大鱼际平面。

【按摩手法】一手持小儿手，使掌心向上，用另一手拇指指腹揉小儿大鱼际。

【功效作用】清胃热，止吐泻，退虚热。

揉外劳宫

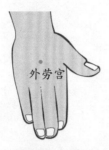

外劳宫

【准确定位】掌背正中，与内劳宫相对处。

【按摩手法】一手握小儿手，使掌背向上，用另一手中指指端揉小儿本穴。

【功效作用】温阳散寒，升阳举陷，发汗解表。

揉一窝风

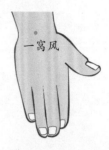

一窝风

【准确定位】腕背侧横纹正中凹陷处。

【按摩手法】一手握小儿手，使掌背向上，用另一手拇指指端揉小儿本穴。

【功效作用】温中行气，疏风解表。

揉二人上马

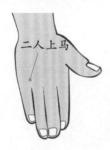

二人上马

【准确定位】手背无名指与小指掌指关节后凹陷中。

【按摩手法】用双手拇指、中指相对按揉小儿本穴。

【功效作用】引火归原，补肾利水，顺气散结。

清补脾经

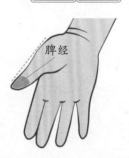

脾经

【准确定位】拇指桡侧缘或拇指末节螺纹面。

【按摩手法】将小儿拇指伸直，循拇指桡侧边缘，由指尖直推到指根，再由指根直推到指尖，如此往返推。

【功效作用】健脾和胃，消食化积。

胃热呕吐

【症状表现】烦躁口渴，腹内热，恶心，食入即吐，吐物酸腐，大便臭秽或见秘结，唇赤，舌质红，苔黄，脉象滑数有力。

【治疗原则】清胃，和中，降逆。

【按摩频率】每天1~2次，直至痊愈。

1. 清肝经5分钟：

用拇指指腹从食指掌面指根直推至指尖。

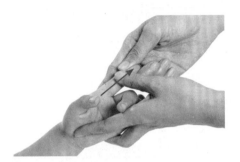

2. 清天河水5分钟：

用食指和中指指腹自掌侧腕横纹推向肘横纹。

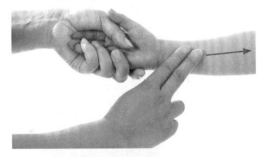

3. 运八卦5分钟：

用拇指指腹自乾宫起顺时针做运法。

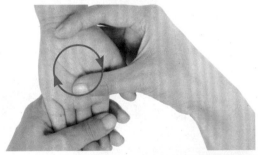

4. 清胃经5分钟：

用拇指指腹从拇指掌根推至拇指指根。

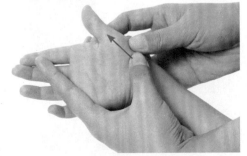

5. 腹痛，加揉板门5分钟：

用拇指指腹揉大鱼际。

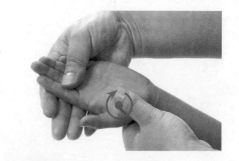

6. 便秘，加清大肠经
5分钟：

用拇指指腹推食指桡侧，由
虎口直推至食指指尖。

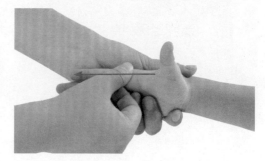

胃寒呕吐

【症状表现】生冷瓜果食用过多，寒滞中脘，或感冷邪，客于胃肠，以
致胃寒上逆，吐物无腐气，腹多寒痛，舌淡苔白，脉弦迟或沉紧。
【治疗原则】温中降逆，驱除寒积。
【按摩频率】每天2次，直至痊愈。

1. 揉外劳宫5分钟：

用中指指端揉掌背正中与内
劳宫相对处。

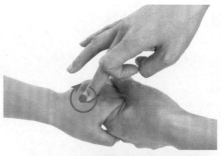

2. 揉板门5分钟：

用拇指指腹揉大鱼际。

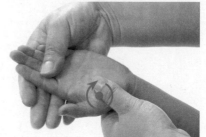

3. ○ 运八卦5分钟：

用拇指指腹自乾宫起顺时针做运法。

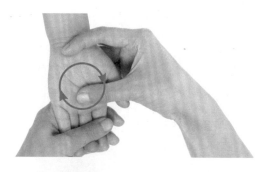

4. ○ 外中寒邪兼腹痛，加揉一窝风5分钟：

用拇指指端揉腕背侧横纹正中凹陷处。

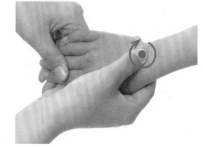

5. ○ 有形寒邪积滞，加清大肠经5分钟：

用拇指指腹推食指桡侧，由虎口直推至指尖。

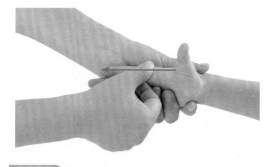

6. ○ 寒伤脾胃或兼冷泻，加清补脾经5分钟：

用拇指指腹循拇指桡侧缘，从指根到指尖来回推。

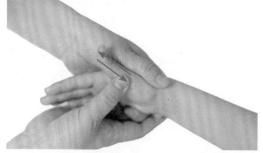

🖐 伤食呕吐

【症状表现】乳儿喂乳过量，或过食甜腻食物及难消化食物，食滞积于中脘，喂乳中忽然呕吐，或见喷溢状呕吐，舌苔厚，脉弦滑。

【治疗原则】消积，降逆止吐。

【按摩频率】每天2次，直至痊愈。

1. 清胃经5分钟：

用拇指指腹从拇指掌根推至拇指指根。

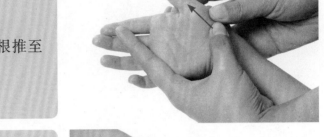

2. 清补脾经5分钟：

用拇指指腹循拇指桡侧缘，从指根到指尖来回推。

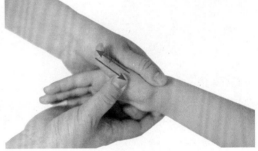

3. 揉板门5分钟：

用拇指指腹揉大鱼际。

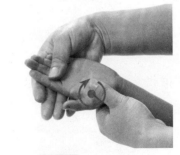

4. 运八卦5分钟：

用拇指指腹自乾宫起顺时针做运法。

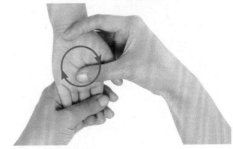

阴虚呕吐

【症状表现】病伤气阴、热耗胃津，胃不得濡，不能润降。表现为厌食、呃逆干呕，食则胃燥不受，反见呕吐，胃阴更耗，必生内热，又称虚火呕吐。

【治疗原则】清补脾胃，降逆止呕。

【按摩频率】每天2次，直至痊愈。

1. 揉二人上马5分钟：

用拇指、中指相对用力揉无名指及小指掌指关节后凹陷处。

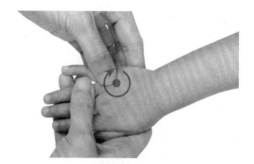

2. 揉板门5分钟：

用拇指指腹揉大鱼际。

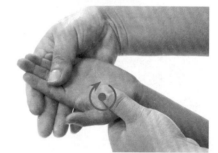

3. 清胃经5分钟：

用拇指指腹自拇指掌根推至拇指指根。

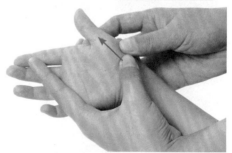

4. 运八卦5分钟：

用拇指指腹自乾宫起顺时针做运法。

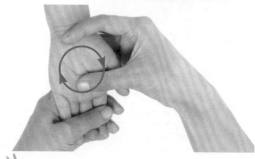

5. 清补脾经5分钟：

用拇指指腹循拇指桡侧缘，从指根到指尖来回推。

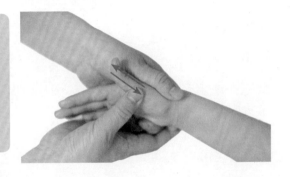

🖐 夹惊呕吐

【症状表现】跌仆受惊，或食时被惊，食随气逆，未见痉挛喷射性呕吐。或痰热上涌，气血逆乱，蛔虫不安上扰，有时吐蛔，皆属此类。必见恶心时作，呕吐黏涎，夜眠多惊，抽搐蠕动，易成惊风。

【治疗原则】平肝镇惊，清热降逆，化痰止咳。

【按摩频率】每天1~2次，直至痊愈。

1. 清肝经5分钟：

用拇指指腹从食指掌面指根直推至指尖。

2. 清胃经5分钟：

用拇指指腹从拇指掌根推至拇指指根。

3. 运八卦5分钟：

用拇指指腹自乾宫起顺时针做运法。

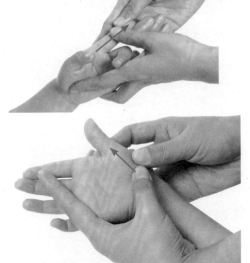

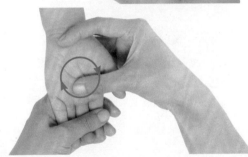

4. ○ 揉板门5分钟：

用拇指指腹揉大鱼际。

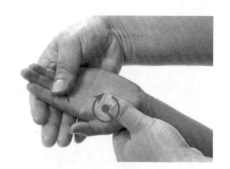

5. ○ 清天河水5分钟：

用食指和中指指腹自腕掌侧横纹推向肘横纹。

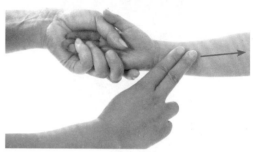

6. ○ 揉外劳宫5分钟：

用中指指端揉掌背正中与内劳宫相对处。

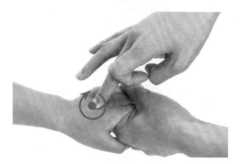

贴心提示

　　如果呕吐不伴有恶心，呈喷射状，伴有头痛、颈部僵硬、精神状态异常或头部曾受过外伤，可能与神经系统伤病有关；如果婴儿哭闹不安，腹胀如鼓，呕吐物有粪臭味，则怀疑肠梗阻；如果婴幼儿出现嗜睡或极度不安，囟门膨出，则是脑膜炎的征象。如有以上情况一定要立刻就诊。

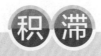

积 滞

　　积滞是指小儿伤于乳食，积滞停留体内不消化而形成的一种脾胃病症，也是消化不良的一种表现。一年四季均可发病，夏秋季节发病率略高，任何年龄段儿童都可患此病，但以婴幼儿为多见。积滞主要表现为不思乳食，食而不化，呕吐，大便不调，腹部胀满，形体瘦弱等。治疗原则以调节脾胃、补充气血为主，兼顾清热除烦。

手部穴位精解

清大肠经

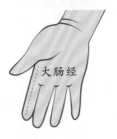

大肠经

揉板门

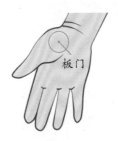

板门

【准确定位】食指桡侧缘，自食指尖到虎口成一直线。

【按摩手法】一手托住小儿手，露出食指桡侧缘，用另一手拇指指腹由小儿虎口直推至指尖。

【功效作用】清利大肠，除湿热。

【准确定位】手掌大鱼际处。

【按摩手法】一手持小儿手，使掌心向上，用另一手拇指指腹揉小儿大鱼际。

【功效作用】清胃热，止吐泻，退虚热。

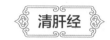

推三关

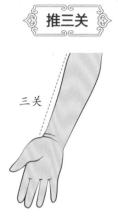

三关

【准确定位】在前臂桡侧，阳池至曲池成一直线。

【按摩手法】一手托住小儿手腕，用另一手食指、中指指腹从小儿手腕推向肘部。

【功效作用】补肾回阳，补虚散寒。

清肝经

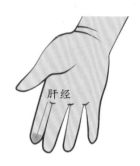

肝经

【准确定位】食指掌面。

【按摩手法】一手托住小儿手，使掌心向上，用另一手拇指指腹从小儿食指指根直推至指尖。

【功效作用】降温，排毒。

补肾经

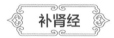

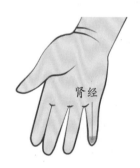

肾经

【准确定位】小指末节螺纹面。

【按摩手法】一手托住小儿手，用另一手拇指指腹旋推小儿小指末节螺纹面。

【功效作用】补肾益脑，温养下焦。

揉外劳宫

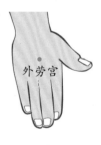

外劳宫

【准确定位】掌背正中，与内劳宫相对处。

【按摩手法】一手握小儿手，使掌背向上，用另一手中指指端揉小儿本穴。

【功效作用】温阳散寒，升阳举陷，发汗解表。

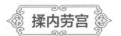

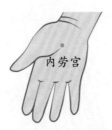

内劳宫

准确定位：在掌心，握拳屈指时中指尖处。

按摩手法：一手握小儿手，使掌心向上，用另一手拇指或中指指端揉小儿本穴。

功效作用：清热除烦，疏风解表。

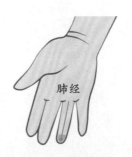

肺经

准确定位：无名指掌面。

按摩手法：一手托住小儿手，使掌心向上，用另一手拇指指腹从小儿无名指指根直推至指尖。

功效作用：宣肺清热，疏风解表，化痰止咳。

运八卦

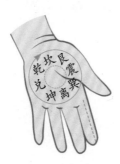

乾坎艮震巽
兑坤离

【**准确定位**】掌中，围绕掌心内劳宫一周，按乾、坎、艮、震、巽、离、坤、兑八卦分布。

【**按摩手法**】一手托住小儿手，使掌心向上，用另一手拇指指腹自小儿乾宫起顺时针做运法。

【**功效作用**】宽胸利膈，理气化痰，行滞消食。

咳嗽痰喘型

【症状表现】不思乳食，食而不化，咳嗽痰喘。

【治疗原则】清热止咳，宽胸理气。

【按摩频率】每天1~2次，10天为1个疗程。

1. 清肺经5分钟：

用拇指指腹从无名指掌面指根直推至指尖。

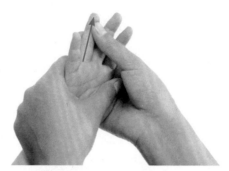

2. 运八卦5分钟：

用拇指指腹自乾宫起顺时针做运法。

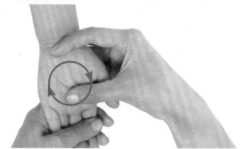

便秘型

【症状表现】脘腹胀满、烦闹啼哭、小便黄或如米泔、大便气味臭秽。

【治疗原则】健脾和胃，泻热通便。

【按摩频率】每天1~2次，10天为1个疗程。

1. 清大肠经5分钟：

用拇指指腹推食指桡侧，由虎口直推至食指指尖。

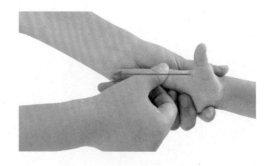

2. 揉板门5分钟：

用拇指指腹揉大鱼际。

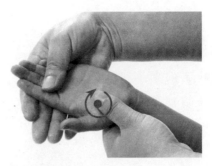

3. 推三关5分钟：

用食指、中指指腹推前臂桡侧，自阳池至曲池。

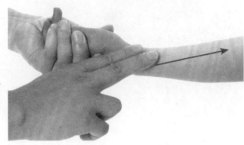

五心烦热型

【症状表现】烦躁不安、眼睛发红、流泪、手脚潮热、睡着后出汗（盗汗）。

【治疗原则】和中清热，消积导滞。

【按摩频率】每天1～2次，10天为1个疗程。

1. 清肝经5分钟：

用拇指指腹从食指掌面指根直推至指尖。

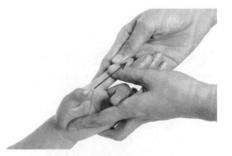

2. 补肾经5分钟：

用拇指指腹旋推小指末节螺纹面。

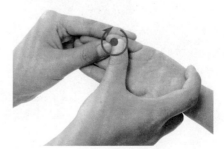

3. 揉内劳宫5分钟：

用拇指指端揉掌心内劳宫。

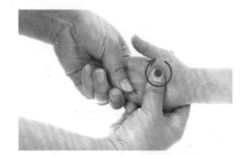

4. 揉外劳宫5分钟：

用中指指端揉掌背正中与内劳宫相对处。

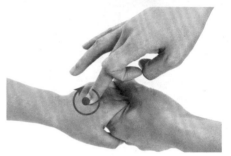

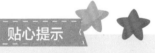
贴心提示

伤食积滞患儿应暂时控制饮食，推拿配合药物调理，待积滞消除后，让患儿逐渐恢复正常饮食。

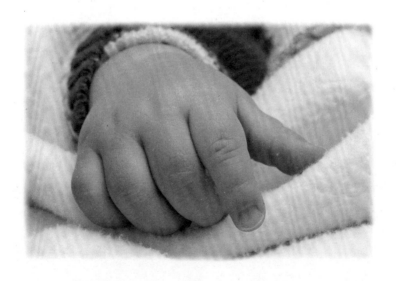

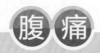

腹痛

　　腹痛是小儿比较常见的病症之一，是多种疾病的常见症状。造成小儿腹痛的原因较多，感受寒邪、乳食积滞、脏腑虚冷、气滞血瘀、蛔虫扰动以及饮食不规律、不卫生等都可引起小儿腹痛。治疗原则以温中散寒、消食导滞为主。

手部穴位精解

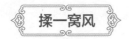

揉一窝风

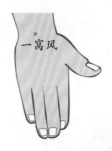

一窝风

【准确定位】腕背侧横纹正中凹陷处。

【按摩手法】一手握小儿手，使掌背向上，用另一手拇指指端揉小儿本穴。

【功效作用】温中行气，疏风解表。

揉外劳宫

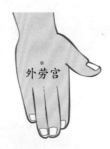

外劳宫

【准确定位】掌背正中，与内劳宫相对处。

【按摩手法】一手握小儿手，使掌背向上，用另一手中指指端揉小儿本穴。

【功效作用】温阳散寒，升阳举陷，发汗解表。

揉板门

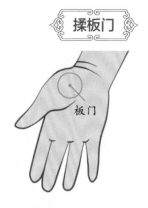

板门

【准确定位】手掌大鱼际处。

【按摩手法】一手持小儿手，使掌心向上，用另一手拇指指腹揉小儿大鱼际。

【功效作用】清胃热，止吐泻，退虚热。

运八卦

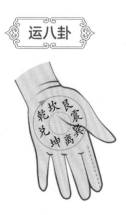

乾 坎 艮 震 巽 离 坤 兑

【准确定位】掌中，围绕掌心内劳宫一周，按乾、坎、艮、震、巽、离、坤、兑八卦分布。

【按摩手法】一手托住小儿手，使掌心向上，用另一手拇指指腹自小儿乾宫起顺时针做运法。

【功效作用】宽胸利膈，理气化痰，行滞消食。

清肝经

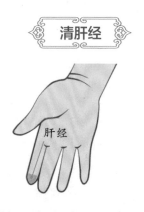

肝经

【准确定位】食指掌面。

【按摩手法】一手托住小儿手，使掌心向上，用另一手拇指指腹从小儿食指指根直推至指尖。

【功效作用】清热，排毒。

清天河水

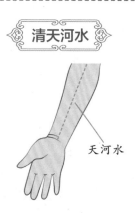

天河水

【准确定位】前臂内侧正中，总筋至洪池成一直线。

【按摩手法】一手握住小儿手，使掌心向上，用另一手食指和中指指腹自小儿腕横纹推向肘横纹。

【功效作用】清心除烦，镇惊安神，退热发表。

清胃经

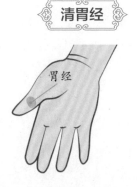

【准确定位】拇指掌面近掌端第一节。

【按摩手法】一手托住小儿手，使掌心向上，用另一手拇指指腹从小儿拇指掌根推至拇指指根。

【功效作用】清胃热，降胃气。

清补脾经

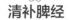
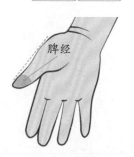

【准确定位】拇指桡侧缘或拇指末节螺纹面。

【按摩手法】将小儿拇指伸直，循拇指桡侧边缘，由指尖直推至指根，再由指根直推至指尖，如此往返推。

【功效作用】健脾和胃，消食化积。

清大肠经

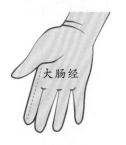

【准确定位】食指桡侧缘，自指尖到虎口成一直线。

【按摩手法】一手托住小儿手，露出食指桡侧缘，用另一手拇指指腹由小儿虎口直推至食指指尖。

【功效作用】清利大肠，除湿热。

推四横纹

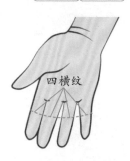

【准确定位】掌面食指、中指、无名指、小指第一指间关节横纹处。

【按摩手法】一手持小儿手，使掌心向上，用另一手拇指指腹从小儿食指横纹推向小指横纹处，来回推。

【功效作用】调中行气，和气血，消胀满。

🖐 寒性腹痛

【症状表现】感受寒邪，脐腹为风寒所侵；或当风进食，或恣食瓜果生冷，寒邪滞于胃肠，寒凝收引，不能通和，因而作痛。痛多绕脐，思热饮，喜暖熨，舌苔薄白，脉象沉紧或迟。

【治疗原则】温中散寒，理气止痛。

【按摩频率】每天2次，至症状缓解。

1. 揉一窝风5分钟：

用拇指指端揉腕背侧横纹正中凹陷处。

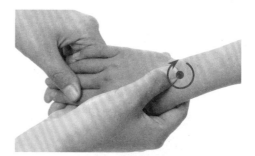

2. 揉外劳宫5分钟：

用中指指端揉掌背正中与内劳宫相对处。

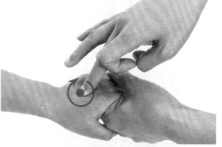

3. 揉板门5分钟：

用拇指指腹揉大鱼际。

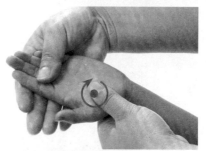

4. 清天河水5分钟：

用食指和中指指腹自腕掌侧横纹推至肘横纹。

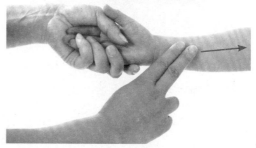

5. 有形寒积者，加清补
大肠经5分钟：

用拇指指腹来回推孩子食
指桡侧缘。

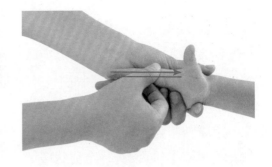

热性腹痛

【症状表现】腹痛，腹外扪之亦热，肠鸣作呕，舌苔黄腻，脉滑濡而数。

【治疗原则】散热，和胃肠，止痛。

【按摩频率】每天2次，至症状缓解。

1. 清肝经5分钟：

用拇指指腹从食指掌面指根
直推至指尖。

2. 清胃经5分钟：

用拇指指腹自拇指掌根推至
拇指指根。

3. 清天河水5分钟：

用食指和中指指腹自腕掌侧
横纹推至肘横纹。

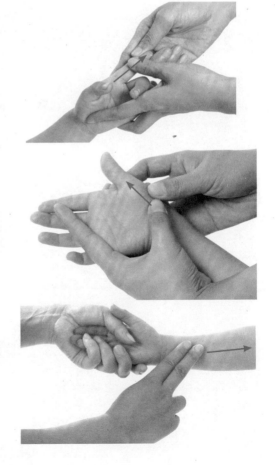

4. 揉板门5分钟：

用拇指指腹揉大鱼际。

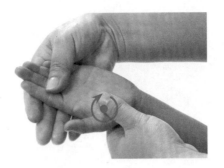

🖐 食积腹痛

【症状表现】饮食不节、零食无度、食积不消，最易生热。症见肠鸣辘辘，扪之有散块，或见呕吐，得泻痛减，苔厚，脉滑数。

【治疗原则】消导，清热，止痛。

【按摩频率】每天2次，至症状缓解。

1. 清肝经5分钟：

用拇指指腹从食指掌面指根直推至指尖。

2. 清胃经5分钟：

用拇指指腹自拇指掌根推至拇指指根。

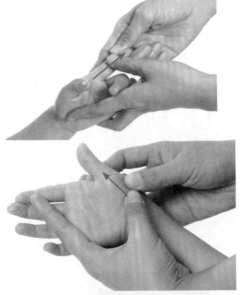

3. 揉板门5分钟：

用拇指指腹揉大鱼际。

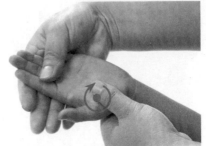

4. 清大肠经5分钟：

用拇指指腹推食指桡侧，
由虎口直推至食指指尖。

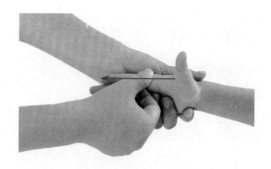

气郁腹痛

【症状表现】小孩因故哭叫，家人抑制使其不能发泄，或强以乳食，迫使小儿止哭入睡，睡中时作痉挛性长息，易患胸胁痛，甚至发热，一般皆以为腹痛，以痛时身体扭动为特征，或见呃逆，舌苔滞（舌苔与舌质不能分离），脉弦紧。

【治疗原则】理气止痛。

【按摩频率】每天2次，至症状缓解。

1. 清肝经5分钟：

用拇指指腹从食指掌面指根
直推至指尖。

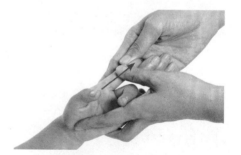

2. 运八卦5分钟：

用拇指指腹自乾宫起顺时针
做运法。

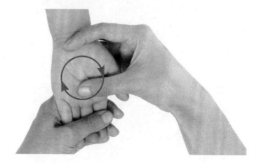

3. 推四横纹5分钟：

用拇指指腹从食指横纹推向小指横纹，来回推。

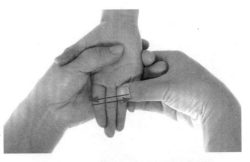

4. 揉板门5分钟：

用拇指指腹揉大鱼际。

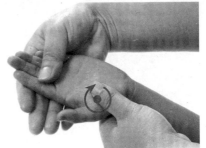

瘀血腹痛

【症状表现】小儿跌仆较重，时见微热，痛在胸腹，痛时身体不动或少动，印堂青，舌偏青黯，脉紧涩。

【治疗原则】活血化瘀，止痛。

【按摩频率】每天2次，至症状缓解。

1. 推四横纹5分钟：

用拇指指腹从食指横纹推向小指横纹，来回推。

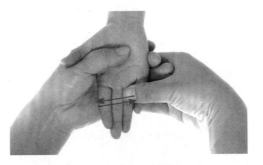

2. 揉外劳宫5分钟：

用中指指端揉掌背正中与内劳宫相对处。

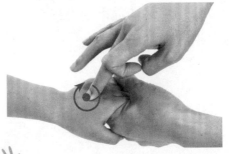

3. ○ 揉板门5分钟：

用拇指指腹揉大鱼际。

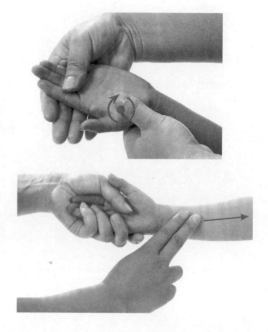

4. ○ 清天河水5分钟：

用食指和中指指腹自腕掌侧横纹推至肘横纹。

虚寒腹痛

【症状表现】小儿倦怠纳呆，四肢无力，时见厥冷，睡时俯身而卧，正之仍俯，眠中露睛，腹部喜按喜热熨，实为慢性隐痛而患儿不能自诉，面色苍白，舌苔淡薄白，脉沉紧，久成慢惊。

【治疗原则】温中，健脾，止痛。

【按摩频率】每天2次，至症状缓解。

1. ○ 揉外劳宫5分钟：

用中指指端揉掌背正中与内劳宫相对处。

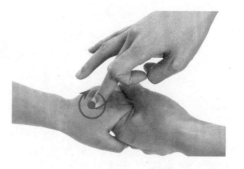

2. 清补脾经5分钟：

用拇指指腹循拇指桡侧缘，从指根到指尖来回推。

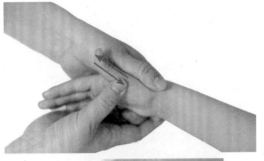

3. 揉板门5分钟：

用拇指指腹揉大鱼际。

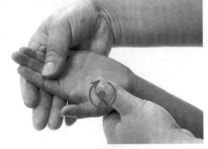

4. 推四横纹5分钟：

用拇指指腹从食指横纹推向小指横纹处，来回推。

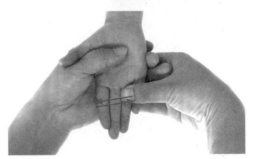

 贴心提示

　　肠套叠腹痛：患儿不进食也腹痛，大便闭，腹肌紧张，舌色淡，脉沉细涩。需立即就医。

　　蛔虫症腹痛：痛时上身扭动，下唇内黏膜扪之如沙砾状。小儿好挖鼻孔，时或吐蛔。需就医。

　　剧烈或持续腹痛患儿应卧床休息，并做必要的辅助检查，对于肠套叠腹痛、蛔虫症腹痛或其他不明原因引起的腹痛，应及时就医。

腹 泻

　　腹泻是指大便次数增多，粪质稀薄，甚至如水样的一种病症。腹泻是小儿常见病，多见于6个月至2岁的婴幼儿，一年四季均可发病，但以夏、秋季多见。轻微的腹泻痊愈较快，但如果腹泻症状重，病程长，则耗伤小儿津液，导致疳病，甚至慢惊风。中医认为，小儿腹泻分为积泻、惊泻、伤泻、冷泻、热泻等多种证型，主要病因为内伤乳食、感受外邪和脾胃虚弱。治疗原则以温中、清热、健脾为主。

手部穴位精解

揉外劳宫

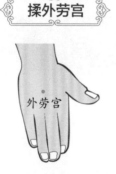

外劳宫

清胃经

胃经

【准确定位】掌背正中，与内劳宫相对处。

【按摩手法】一手握住小儿手，使掌背向上，用另一手中指指端揉小儿本穴。

【功效作用】温阳散寒，升阳举陷，发汗解表。

【准确定位】拇指掌面近掌端第一节。

【按摩手法】一手托住小儿手，使掌心向上，用另一手拇指指腹从小儿拇指掌根推至拇指指根。

【功效作用】清胃热，降胃气。

清天河水

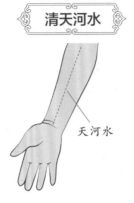

天河水

【准确定位】前臂内侧正中，总筋至洪池成一直线。

【按摩手法】一手握住小儿手，使掌心向上，用另一手食指和中指指腹自小儿腕横纹推向肘横纹。

【功效作用】清心除烦，镇惊安神，退热发表。

退六腑

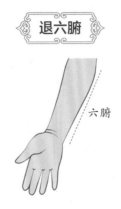

六腑

【准确定位】前臂尺侧，肘至阴池成一直线。

【按摩手法】一手握住小儿手腕，用另一手食指、中指指腹自小儿肘横纹尺侧端推至腕掌侧横纹尺侧端。

【功效作用】清热解毒，消肿止痛。

清大肠经

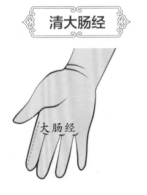

大肠经

【准确定位】食指桡侧缘，自食指尖到虎口成一直线。

【按摩手法】一手托住小儿手，露出食指桡侧缘，用另一手拇指指腹由小儿虎口直推至食指指尖。

【功效作用】清利大肠，除湿热。

清脾经

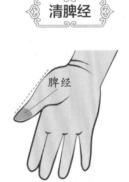

脾经

【准确定位】拇指桡侧缘或拇指末节螺纹面。

【按摩手法】一手持小儿手掌，使掌心向上，用另一手将小儿拇指伸直，沿拇指桡侧缘，自指根直推至指尖。

【功效作用】健脾胃，清热利湿。

运八卦

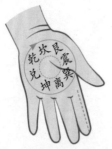

【准确定位】掌中，围绕掌心内劳宫一周，按乾、坎、艮、震、巽、离、坤、兑八卦分布。

【按摩手法】一手托住小儿手，使掌心向上，用另一手拇指指腹自小儿乾宫起顺时针做运法。

【功效作用】宽胸利膈，理气化痰，行滞消食。

清肝经

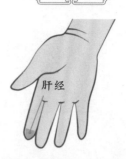

【准确定位】食指掌面。

【按摩手法】一手托住小儿手，使掌心向上，用另一手拇指指腹从小儿食指指根直推至指尖。

【功效作用】降温，排毒。

清小肠经

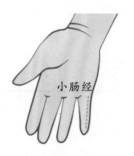

【准确定位】小指尺侧缘，自指尖至指根成一直线。

【按摩手法】一手托住小儿手，使掌心向上，另一手拇指指腹从小儿小指尺侧指根推到指尖。

【功效作用】清利下焦湿热。

揉二人上马

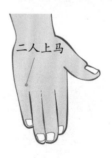

【准确定位】手背无名指与小指掌指关节后凹陷中。

【按摩手法】用双手拇指、中指相对用力按揉小儿本穴。

【功效作用】引火归原，补肾利水，顺气散结。

寒湿腹泻

【症状表现】腹痛肠鸣，泄泻清澈，白水泻或色绿，小便清白，面色淡白。

【治疗原则】温中止泻。

【按摩频率】每天1次，至症状缓解。

1. 揉外劳宫20分钟：

用中指指端揉掌背正中与内劳宫相对处。

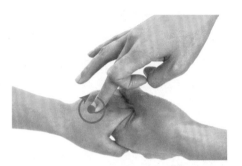

2. 清胃经5分钟：

用拇指指腹自拇指掌根推至拇指指根。

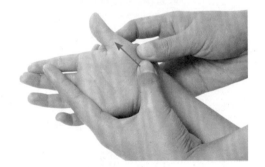

3. 清天河水5分钟：

用食指和中指指腹自腕掌侧横纹推至肘横纹。

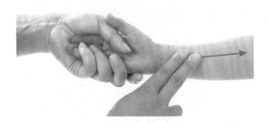

湿热腹泻

【症状表现】泻时暴注下迫、大便色黄赤、泻多黄水、有热臭、口渴烦躁、腹痛身热、溲少而黄、肛门灼热。

【治疗原则】清热止泻。

【按摩频率】每天1次，至症状缓解。

1. 退六腑5分钟：

用食指、中指指腹自肘部尺侧推向手腕尺侧。

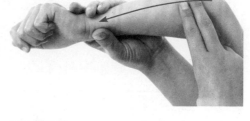

2. 清大肠经5分钟：

用拇指指腹推食指桡侧，由虎口直推至食指指尖。

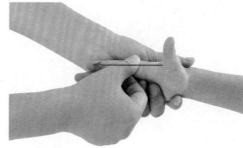

3. 清脾经5分钟：

用拇指指腹循拇指桡侧缘，从指根推向指尖。

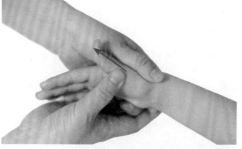

4. 清胃经5分钟：

用拇指指腹自拇指掌根推至拇指指根。

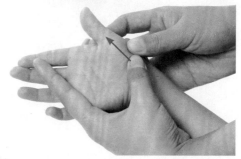

脾虚腹泻

【症状表现】食后作泻，消化不良，大便溏，色淡黄，重则完谷不化，腹胀不渴，面黄肌瘦，不思饮食等。

【治疗原则】健脾止泻。

【按摩频率】每天1次，至症状缓解。

1. 清肝经5分钟：

用拇指指腹从食指掌面指根直推至指尖。

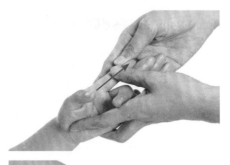

2. 清补脾经5分钟：

用拇指指腹循拇指桡侧缘，从指根到指尖来回推。

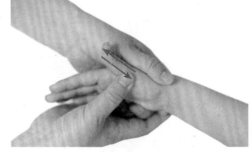

3. 揉外劳宫5分钟：

用中指指端揉掌背正中与内劳宫相对处。

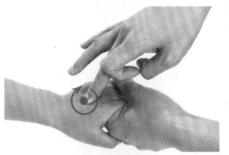

4. 揉二人上马5分钟：

用拇指、中指指腹相对用力揉手背无名指及小指掌指关节后凹陷处。

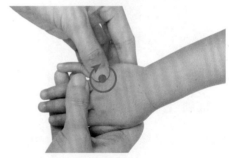

伤食腹泻

【症状表现】口嗳酸气，口渴恶食，腹热胀满，泻时腹痛，泻后痛减，小便赤涩，大便色黄白，臭如败卵，或呕吐。伤乳泻者，大便色黄白，内有奶瓣或呈蛋花样。

【治疗原则】健脾助运化，止泻。

1. 运八卦5分钟：

用拇指指腹自乾宫起顺时针做运法。

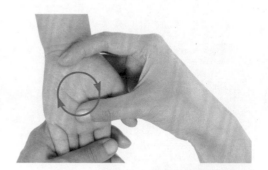

2. 清胃经5分钟：

用拇指指腹自拇指掌根推至拇指指根。

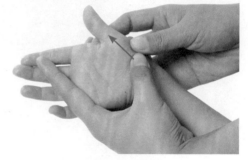

3. 清天河水5分钟：

用食指和中指指腹自腕掌侧横纹推至肘横纹。

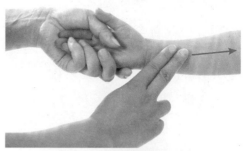

4. 清小肠经5分钟：

用拇指指腹从小指尺侧指根推到指尖。

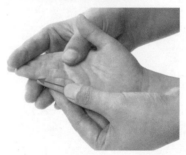

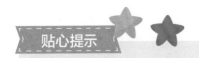

贴心提示

　　小儿腹泻，尤其是婴儿，容易发生脱水，危险性很高。脱水的征象有口渴显著，尿少或呈深黄色，口干，眼窝下陷，皮肤失去正常弹性。如果腹泻伴有发热，粪便为黏液血便或脓血便，频繁水泻，粪便带血或为黑粪，腹泻伴有剧烈腹痛，往往意味着较严重的病症，应尽快前往医院就医。对痢疾或可能导致严重脱水的腹泻要及时就医。

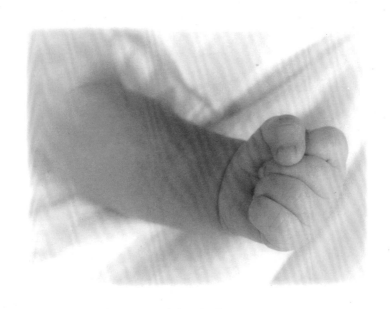

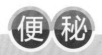

便秘是指大便干燥坚硬、排便次数减少、间隔时间延长或大便排出困难的一种病症。中医认为婴幼儿便秘的发生，多由于气滞不行、气虚传导无力，或病后体虚，津液耗伤，肠道干涩等原因导致大肠传导功能失常，粪便在肠内停留太久，水分被吸收，从而使粪质过于干燥、坚硬。治疗原则以健脾行气、清泄里热、导滞通便为主。

手部穴位精解

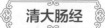

清大肠经

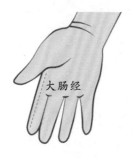

大肠经

【准确定位】食指桡侧缘，自食指尖到虎口成一直线。

【按摩手法】一手托住小儿手，露出食指桡侧缘，用另一手拇指指腹由小儿虎口直推至指尖。

【功效作用】清利大肠，除湿热。

清肝经

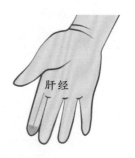

肝经

【准确定位】食指掌面。

【按摩手法】一手托住小儿手，使掌心向上，用另一手拇指指腹从小儿食指指根直推至指尖。

【功效作用】清热，排毒。

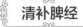

清补脾经

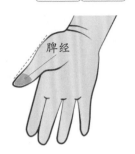

脾经

【准确定位】拇指桡侧缘或拇指末节螺纹面。

【按摩手法】将小儿拇指伸直，循拇指桡侧边缘，由指尖直推到指根，再由指根直推到指尖，如此往返推。

【功效作用】健脾和胃，消食化积。

推四横纹

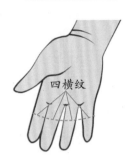

四横纹

【准确定位】掌面食指、中指、无名指、小指第一指间关节横纹处。

【按摩手法】一手持小儿手，使掌心向上，用另一手拇指指腹从小儿食指横纹推向小指横纹处，来回推。

【功效作用】调中行气，和气血，消胀满。

清天河水

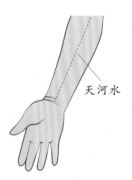

天河水

【准确定位】前臂内侧正中，总筋至洪池成一直线。

【按摩手法】一手握住小儿手，使掌心向上，用另一手食指和中指指腹自小儿腕横纹推向肘横纹。

【功效作用】清心除烦，镇惊安神，退热发表。

实秘型便秘

【症状表现】大便秘结、排便费力、几日一行，重者肛裂出血或脱肛。

【治疗原则】健脾行气，清泄里热，导滞通便。

【按摩频率】每天1次，5天为1个疗程。

1. 清补脾经5分钟：

用拇指指腹循拇指桡侧缘，从指根到指尖来回推。

2. 清大肠经5分钟：

用拇指指腹推食指桡侧，由虎口直推至食指指尖。

3. 运水入土5分钟：

用左手拇指、中指捏住小儿拇指，使其掌心向上，用右手拇指指腹循小儿小指掌面尺侧缘→小鱼际尺侧缘→腕掌侧横纹→大鱼际桡侧缘→拇指掌面桡侧缘→拇指指端做运法。

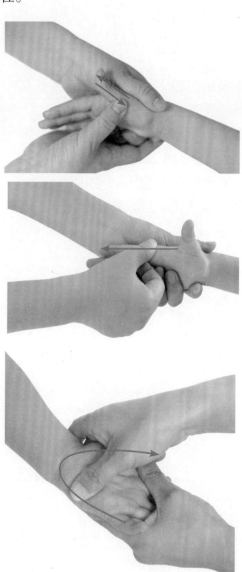

4. 清肝经5分钟：

用拇指指腹从食指掌面指根直推至指尖。

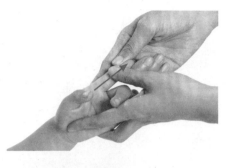

5. 便秘伴发热时，清天河水3分钟：

用食指和中指指腹自腕掌侧横纹推至肘横纹。

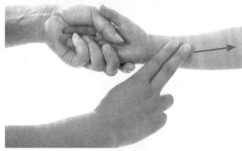

6. 推四横纹5分钟：

用拇指指腹从食指横纹推向小指横纹处，来回推。

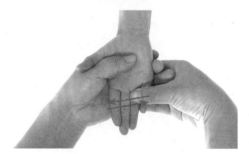

食疗小偏方

莱菔子散：

　　取莱菔子适量，炒黄，研成细末，装瓶备用。每次取5～10克用温蜂蜜水冲服。适用于食积便秘。

润肠散：

　　取南瓜子、松子、黑芝麻、花生仁、白糖各等量，将南瓜子与松子炒香，去壳，将黑芝麻与花生仁炒香，与去壳的南瓜子与松子一同研碎，加入白糖。每次1匙，温水送服，每日2～3次。适用于虚秘。

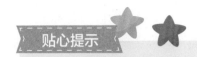

贴心提示

　　不要给孩子随意服用消食通便的中成药，消食通便的中成药适用于胃肠积滞不通的实证，不适用于胃肠动力不足的虚性积食、便秘。消食通便药一般都含有大量的行气、破气中药，虚性积食、便秘者用之，则会损伤脾胃，加重积食、便秘。

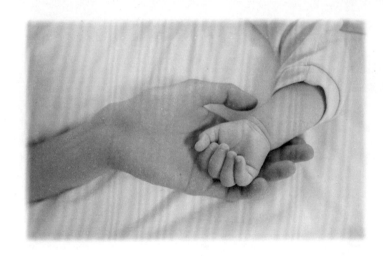

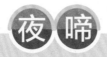

小儿夜啼的表现是每到夜间即高声啼哭，间歇性发作，甚至通宵达旦啼哭不止，白天却安静不哭。此症多见于半岁以下婴儿，孩子一般身体情况良好，与季节无明显关系。如果孩子总在夜晚啼哭，千万不要以为是正常现象而盲目喂食或者只是单纯哄哄孩子。因为长久性的夜间啼哭与身体的不同病症是紧密相连的，最好能针对孩子不同的啼哭特点，经常给孩子做做按摩，缓解这种情况。

✋ 手部穴位精解

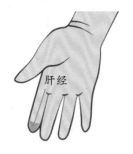

肝经

【准确定位】食指掌面。

【按摩手法】一手托住小儿手，使掌心向上，用另一手拇指指腹从小儿食指指根直推至指尖。

【功效作用】清热，排毒。

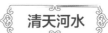

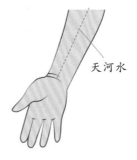

天河水

【准确定位】前臂内侧正中，总筋至洪池成一直线。

【按摩手法】一手握住小儿手，使掌心向上，用另一手食指和中指指腹自小儿腕横纹推向肘横纹。

【功效作用】清心除烦，镇惊安神，退热发表。

清心经

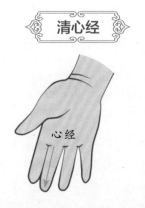

【准确定位】掌面，中指指面。

【按摩手法】一手持小儿手，另一手拇指指腹从小儿中指指根直推至指尖。

【功效作用】清热，退心火。

清小肠经

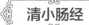
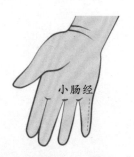

【准确定位】小指尺侧缘，自指尖至指根成一直线。

【按摩手法】一手托住小儿手，另一手拇指指腹从小儿小指尺侧指根推到指尖。

【功效作用】清利下焦湿热。

补脾经

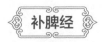
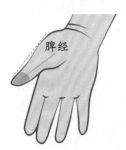

【准确定位】拇指桡侧缘或拇指末节螺纹面。

【按摩手法】一手持小儿小指，用另一手拇指指腹旋推小儿拇指末节螺纹面。

【功效作用】健脾胃，补气血。

补肾经

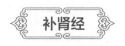
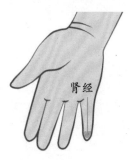

【准确定位】小指末节螺纹面。

【按摩手法】一手托住小儿手，用另一手拇指指腹旋推小儿小指末节螺纹面。

【功效作用】补肾益脑，温养下焦。

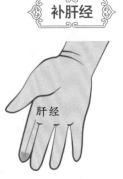

补肝经

【准确定位】食指末节螺纹面。

【按摩手法】一手持小儿食指末节，用另一手拇指指腹旋推小儿食指末节螺纹面。

【功效作用】养血，柔肝。

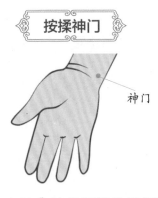

按揉神门

神门

【准确定位】腕掌侧横纹尺侧端凹陷处。

【按摩手法】一手持小儿手，用另一手拇指指端按揉小儿本穴。

【功效作用】补心益气，安神降火。

心火旺型

【症状表现】烦躁不安，面红耳赤，怕见灯光，大便干燥，小便发黄。

【治疗原则】清心泻火，引火归原。

【按摩频率】每天2次。

1. 清肝经5分钟：

用拇指指腹从食指掌面指根直推至指尖。

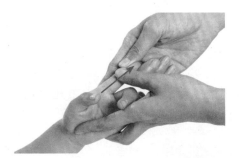

2. 清心经5分钟：

用拇指指腹从中指掌面指根直推至指尖。

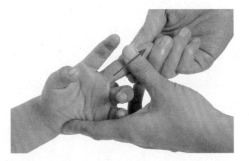

3. 清小肠经3分钟：

用拇指指腹从小指尺侧指根推到指尖。

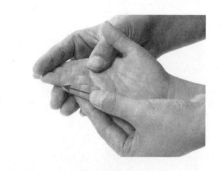

4. 清天河水3分钟：

用食指和中指指腹自腕掌侧横纹推至肘横纹。

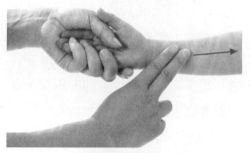

5. 补脾经3分钟：

用拇指指腹旋推拇指末节螺纹面。

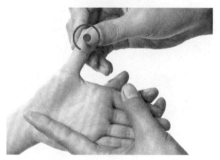

6. 补肾经3分钟：

用拇指指腹旋推小指末节螺纹面。

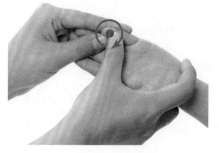

惊恐型

【症状表现】哭声比较惨，心神不安、面色发青，时睡时醒。

【治疗原则】安神镇惊。

【按摩频率】每天2次。

1. 按揉神门3分钟：

用拇指指端按揉腕掌侧横纹尺侧端凹陷处。

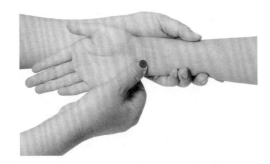

2. 清心经5分钟：

用拇指指腹从中指掌面指根直推至指尖。

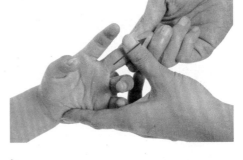

3. 补肝经5分钟：

用拇指指腹旋推食指末节螺纹面。

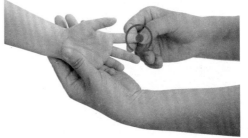

 贴心提示

引起孩子夜间啼哭的原因很多，应先查找生理性原因，如饥饿、尿布潮湿、过冷、过热、衣着不适等。还要警惕病理性原因，如发热、积滞、中耳炎、肠套叠等，家长要注意观察，必要时就医。

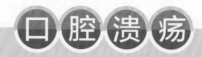

口腔溃疡

　　口腔溃疡，是指牙龈、舌、两颊和上腭等处出现淡黄色或灰白色的溃疡。口疮是一种常见的口腔疾病，经常反复发作，溃疡局部灼热、疼痛，严重的会影响孩子进食。中医认为，口疮是感受外邪，风热乘脾，心脾积热或素体虚弱，虚火上炎所致。治疗原则以补肾滋阴、清心泻火为主。

手部穴位精解

清胃经

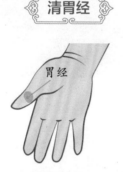

胃经

【准确定位】拇指掌面靠近掌端第一节。

【按摩手法】一手托住小儿手，使掌心向上，用另一手拇指指腹从小儿拇指掌根推至拇指指根。

【功效作用】清胃热，降胃气。

清天河水

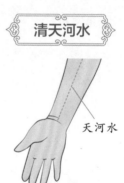

天河水

【准确定位】前臂内侧正中，总筋至洪池成一直线。

【按摩手法】一手握住小儿手，使掌心向上，用另一手食指和中指指腹自小儿腕横纹推向肘横纹。

【功效作用】清心除烦，镇惊安神，退热发表。

推四横纹

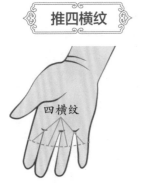

四横纹

【准确定位】掌面食指、中指、无名指、小指第一指间关节横纹处。

【按摩手法】一手持小儿手，使掌心向上，用另一手拇指指腹从小儿食指横纹推向小指横纹处，来回推。

【功效作用】调中行气，和气血，消胀满。

清脾经

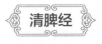

脾经

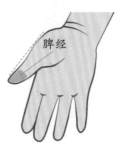

【准确定位】拇指桡侧缘或拇指末节螺纹面。

【按摩手法】一手持小儿手掌，使掌心向上，另一手将小儿拇指伸直，沿拇指桡侧缘，自指根直推至指尖。

【功效作用】健脾胃，清热利湿。

补肾经

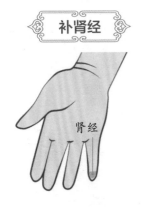

肾经

【准确定位】小指末节螺纹面。

【按摩手法】一手托住小儿手，用另一手拇指指腹旋推小儿小指末节螺纹面。

【功效作用】补肾益脑，温养下焦。

清小肠经

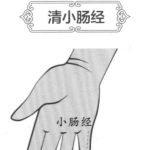

小肠经

【准确定位】小指尺侧缘，自指尖至指根成一直线。

【按摩手法】一手托住小儿手，使掌心向上，另一手拇指指腹从小儿小指尺侧指根推到指尖。

【功效作用】清利下焦湿热。

一般性口腔溃疡

【症状表现】舌尖红赤，舌有白色溃疡，流口水，往往因疼痛而吮乳困难，重者发热，烦躁不安。

【治疗原则】清心泻火，引火归原。

【按摩频率】每天2次。

1. 清脾经5分钟：

用拇指指腹循拇指桡侧缘，从指根推向指尖。

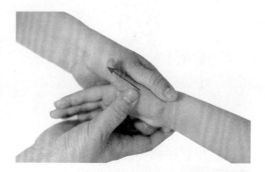

2. 清胃经5分钟：

用拇指指腹自拇指掌根推至拇指指根。

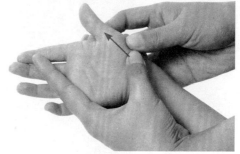

3. 清天河水5分钟：

用食指和中指指腹自腕掌侧横纹推至肘横纹。

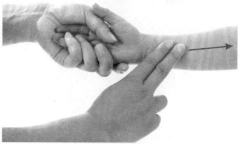

4. 推四横纹5分钟：

用拇指指腹从食指横纹推向小指横纹处，来回推。

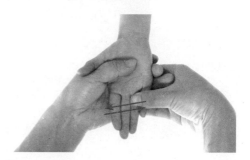

5. ● 补肾经3分钟：

用拇指指腹旋推小指末节螺纹面。

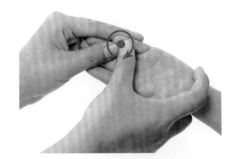

6. ● 清小肠经3分钟：

用拇指指腹从小指尺侧指根推到指尖。

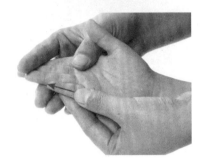

食疗小偏方

荷叶冬瓜汤：

　　鲜荷叶1张，鲜冬瓜500克，盐少许。锅置火上，放入洗好的荷叶、切好的冬瓜（去瓤）、适量清水煲汤，熟后加入盐，饮汤食冬瓜。具有清热解暑、生津止渴、降心火的作用。适用于心火上升的口疮患者，尤其对暑天的实热型口腔炎症效果更佳。

冰糖炖银耳：

　　银耳10～12克，冰糖适量。将银耳洗净放入碗内，加冷开水浸泡1小时左右，以浸透银耳为度，除去杂质。锅置火上，放入银耳、冰糖，用冷开水隔水炖2～3小时，即可服用。具有滋阴生津、润肺、养心阴的作用。适用于虚火上升的口疮患者。

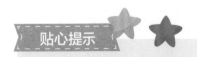 贴心提示

　　如果孩子经常长口疮，即使口疮暂时好了，家长也要按照治疗口疮的按摩手法坚持给孩子按摩1个月，以巩固疗效。此外，不要给孩子吃过热、过硬及刺激性的食物，注意口腔卫生，养成饭后漱口的好习惯。

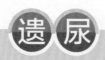

遗 尿

小儿5岁以上如仍在睡眠过程中不自主排尿，称为遗尿。中医认为，遗尿主要与肾和膀胱的气化功能失调有关，也与脾、肺的宣散传输和肝的疏泄失常有关。小儿先天不足或体质较差，肾气不足或脾肺气虚、肝经湿热，都会造成膀胱失约而遗尿。治疗原则以补益肾气、提升阳气为主。

手部穴位精解

清胃经

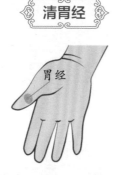

胃经

清天河水

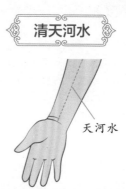

天河水

【准确定位】拇指的掌面近掌端第一节。

【按摩手法】一手托住小儿手，使掌心向上，用另一手拇指指腹从小儿拇指掌根推至拇指指根。

【功效作用】清胃热，降胃气。

【准确定位】前臂内侧正中，总筋至洪池成一直线。

【按摩手法】一手握住小儿手，使掌心向上，用另一手食指和中指指腹自小儿腕横纹推向肘横纹。

【功效作用】清心除烦，镇惊安神，退热发表。

补脾经

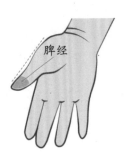

脾经

【准确定位】拇指桡侧缘或拇指末节螺纹面。

【按摩手法】一手持小儿小指，用另一手拇指指腹旋推小儿拇指末节螺纹面。

【功效作用】健脾胃，补气血。

补肾经

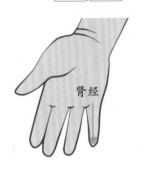

肾经

【准确定位】小指末节螺纹面。

【按摩手法】一手托住小儿手，用另一手拇指指腹旋推小儿小指末节螺纹面。

【功效作用】补肾益脑，温养下焦。

揉二人上马

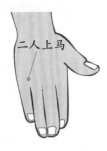

二人上马

【准确定位】手背无名指及小指掌指关节后凹陷中。

【按摩手法】用双手拇指、中指相对用力按揉小儿本穴。

【功效作用】引火归原，补肾利水，顺气散结。

补肺经

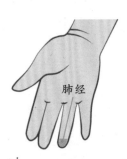

肺经

【准确定位】无名指末节螺纹面。

【按摩手法】一手托住小儿手，使掌心向上，用另一手拇指指腹旋推小儿无名指末节螺纹面。

【功效作用】补益肺气。

肝脏湿热型

【症状表现】夜间遗尿，睡不安宁，尿色黄，尿频而短涩，面色红赤，性情急躁。

【治疗原则】补肺益脾，固涩膀胱。

【按摩频率】每天按摩1次，10天为1个疗程。病程短者，一般1~2个疗程即可治愈，最好再巩固一段时间。病程长者，需要2~3个疗程，症状才能减轻。继续按摩2~3个疗程方可痊愈，以后可改为隔日1次。

1. 清天河水3分钟：

用食指和中指指腹自腕掌侧横纹推至肘横纹。

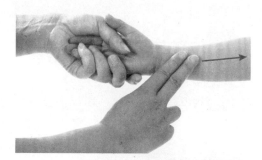

2. 清胃经5分钟：

用拇指指腹自拇指掌根推至拇指指根。

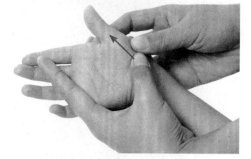

3. 补肾经3分钟：

用拇指指腹旋推小指末节螺纹面。

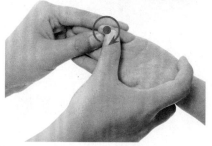

脾肺气虚型

【症状表现】精神疲倦，形体消瘦，大便清稀，食欲不振。

【症状表现】补肺益脾，固涩膀胱。

【按摩频率】每天按摩1次，10天为1个疗程。病程短者，一般1~2个疗程即可治愈，最好再巩固一段时间。病程长者，需要2~3个疗程，症状才能减轻。继续按摩2~3个疗程方可痊愈，以后可改为隔日1次。

1. 补脾经5分钟：

用拇指指腹旋推拇指末节螺纹面。

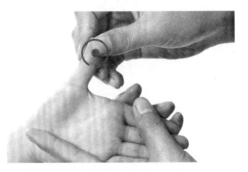

2. 补肺经5分钟：

用拇指指腹旋推无名指末节螺纹面。

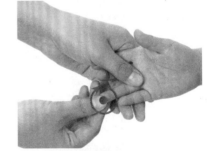

3. 揉二人上马5分钟：

用拇指、中指相对用力揉手背无名指与小指掌指关节后的凹陷处。

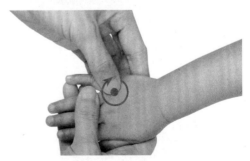

4. 运水入土5分钟：

用左手拇指、中指捏住小儿拇指，使其掌心向上，用右手拇指指腹循小儿小指掌面尺侧缘→小鱼际尺侧缘→腕掌侧横纹→大鱼际桡侧缘→拇指掌面桡侧缘→拇指指端做运法。

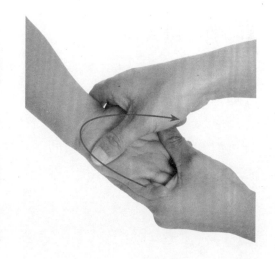

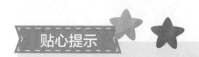

食疗小偏方

小肚汤：

取益智、乌药、小茴香各10克，装入猪肚内，放入砂锅中，加鸡内金10克，一起煮至猪肚烂熟，加入大青盐10克即成。早晚空腹吃猪肚喝汤，连服5次。适用于脾肺气虚型遗尿。

肉苁蓉羊肉粥：

羊肉（瘦）100克，粳米100克，肉苁蓉10克，食盐1克，姜末3克，葱末3克。将肉苁蓉煎汤去渣取汁，加羊肉、粳米同煮做粥，放入食盐、葱末、姜末等调味。属温热性药粥方，适宜冬季服食，5~7天为1个疗程。适用于肾阳虚衰所致的遗尿。

贴心提示

小儿遗尿时心理调护非常重要，不要责骂或讽刺孩子，不要使孩子有心理负担。家长要对患儿进行排尿训练。晚间控制饮水量，临睡前排尿后再就寝，睡觉时定时唤醒孩子排尿。白天要避免孩子过度紧张、兴奋或疲惫。部分孩子遗尿是由泌尿系统疾患所致，应及时就医检查。

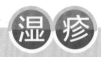

湿疹

　　婴儿湿疹又叫奶癣，是婴儿期常见的皮肤病，经常反复发作，但常在2岁以内自愈。中医认为，湿疹为内蕴湿热，外感热邪，发于肌肤所致。如果母亲怀孕时喜欢吃辛辣燥热的食物或感受湿邪，则湿热会传给胎儿，出生后蕴阻在皮肤而成为湿疹。小儿肌肤娇嫩，容易感受外邪，风、湿、热邪互相搏结，发于皮肤，出现湿疹。如果喂养不当，脾胃运化失职，聚湿生热，发于肌肤也会引起湿疹。治疗原则以清热除湿为主。

手部穴位精解

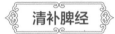

清补脾经

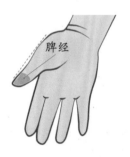

脾经

【准确定位】拇指桡侧缘或拇指末节螺纹面。

【按摩手法】将小儿拇指伸直，循拇指桡侧边缘，由指尖直推到指根，再由指根直推到指尖，如此往返推。

【功效作用】健脾和胃，消食化积。

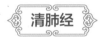

清肺经

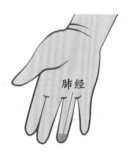

肺经

【准确定位】无名指掌面。

【按摩手法】一手托住小儿手，使掌心向上，用另一手拇指指腹从小儿无名指指根直推至指尖。

【功效作用】宣肺清热，疏风解表，化痰止咳。

补肺经

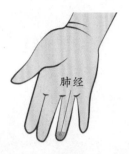

肺经

【准确定位】无名指末节螺纹面。

【按摩手法】一手托住小儿手，使掌心向上，用另一手拇指指腹旋推小儿无名指末节螺纹面。

【功效作用】补益肺气。

清大肠经

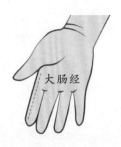

大肠经

【准确定位】食指桡侧缘，从食指指尖到虎口成一直线。

【按摩手法】一手托住小儿手，露出食指桡侧缘，用另一手拇指指腹由小儿虎口直推至食指指尖。

【功效作用】清利大肠，除湿热。

清小肠经

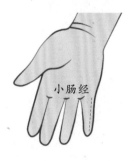

小肠经

【准确定位】小指尺侧缘，自指尖至指根成一直线。

【按摩手法】一手托住小儿手，使掌心向上，另一手拇指指腹从小儿小指尺侧指根推到指尖。

【功效作用】清利下焦湿热。

清天河水

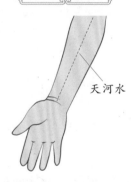

天河水

【准确定位】前臂内侧正中，总筋至洪池成一直线。

【按摩手法】一手握住小儿手，使掌心向上，用另一手食指和中指指腹自小儿腕横纹推向肘横纹。

【功效作用】清心除烦，镇惊安神，退热发表。

普通湿疹

【症状表现】红斑丘疹、水疱、糜烂、渗液等，常对称发于面部、头皮，婴儿湿疹多发生在出生1～6个月，一般在2岁以内可愈。

【治疗原则】清热除湿，祛风止痒。

【按摩频率】每天2次，直至痊愈。

1. 清补脾经5分钟：

用拇指指腹循拇指桡侧缘，从指根到指尖来回推。

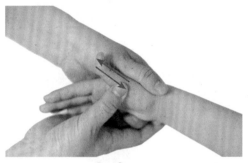

2. 清肺经5分钟：

用拇指指腹从无名指掌面指根直推至指尖。

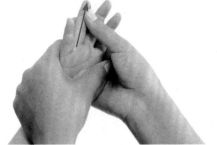

3. 补肺经5分钟：

用拇指指腹旋推无名指末节螺纹面。

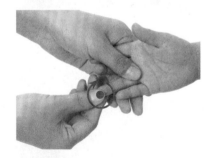

4. 清大肠经5分钟：

用拇指指腹推食指桡侧，由虎口直推至食指指尖。

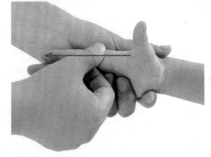

5. 清小肠经5分钟：

用拇指指腹从小指尺侧指根推到指尖。

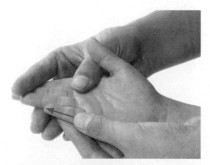

6. 清天河水5分钟：

用食指和中指指腹自腕掌侧横纹推至肘横纹。

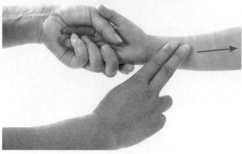

贴心提示 ★ ★

　　湿疹的护理非常重要，患处忌用热水烫洗，忌用肥皂及碱性刺激物，不要使用刺激性强烈的外用药，避免搔抓。急性发作期暂缓预防接种，避免接触单纯疱疹患者。

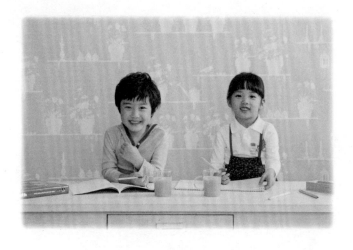

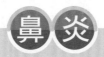

中医称鼻炎为鼻渊，又称脑漏。因其鼻窍不断流涕，犹如泉水，或如黄水，常湿无干，故名鼻渊。其多因外感风热或风寒，肺气虚寒，胆经郁热，郁久化火，上犯于鼻而致。治疗原则以清泻肝胆和宣肺通窍为主。

手部穴位精解

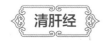

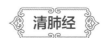

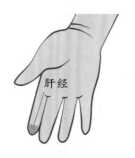

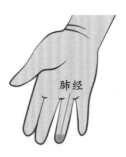

【准确定位】食指掌面。

【按摩手法】一手托住小儿手，使掌心向上，用另一手拇指指腹从小儿食指指根直推至指尖。

【功效作用】清热，排毒。

【准确定位】无名指掌面。

【按摩手法】一手托住小儿手，使掌心向上，用另一手拇指指腹从小儿无名指指根直推至指尖。

【功效作用】宣肺清热，疏风解表，化痰止咳。

揉一窝风

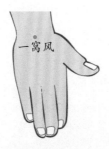

【准确定位】腕背侧横纹正中凹陷处。

【按摩手法】一手握小儿手，使掌背向上，用另一手拇指指端揉小儿本穴。

【功效作用】温中行气，疏风解表。

揉外劳宫

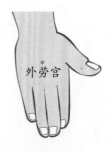

【准确定位】掌背正中，与内劳宫相对处。

【按摩手法】一手握住小儿手，使掌背向上，用另一手中指指端揉小儿本穴。

【功效作用】温阳散寒，升阳举陷，发汗解表。

揉阳池

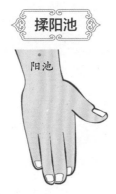

【准确定位】手背一窝风上3寸凹陷处。

【按摩手法】一手握住小儿手腕，使掌背向上，用另一手拇指和中指指端相对用力揉小儿本穴。

【功效作用】降逆，清脑，祛风止痛。

补脾经

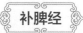
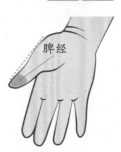

【准确定位】拇指桡侧缘或拇指末节螺纹面。

【按摩手法】一手托住小儿手，用另一手拇指指腹旋推小儿拇指末节螺纹面。

【功效作用】健脾胃，补气血。

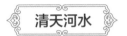

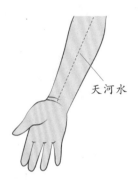

天河水

【准确定位】前臂内侧正中，总筋至洪池成一直线。

【按摩手法】一手握住小儿手，使掌心向上，用另一手食指和中指指腹自小儿腕横纹推向肘横纹。

【功效作用】清心除烦，镇惊安神，退热发表。

寒证

【症状表现】鼻塞，流涕，涕量多，色白、清稀无味，多属寒。

【治疗原则】宣肺通窍。

【按摩频率】每天2次，5天为1个疗程。

1. 补脾经5分钟：

用拇指指腹旋推拇指末节螺纹面。

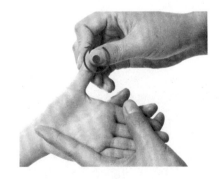

2. ○ 清肺经5分钟：

用拇指指腹从无名指掌面指根直推至指尖。

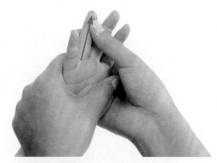

3. ○ 揉一窝风5分钟：

用拇指指端揉腕背侧横纹正中凹陷处。

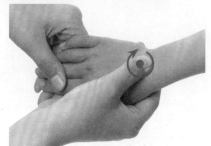

4. ○ 揉外劳宫5分钟：

用中指指端揉掌背正中与内劳宫相对处。

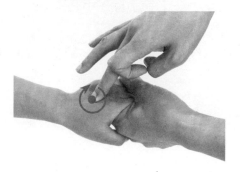

▶ 热证

【症状表现】涕量多，色黄，质稠，有味不重，多属热。

【治疗原则】清泻肝胆。

【按摩频率】每天2次，5天为1个疗程。

1. ○ 清天河水5分钟：

用食指和中指指腹自腕掌侧横纹推至肘横纹。

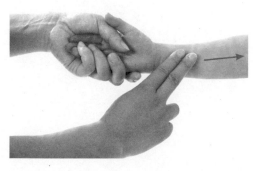

2. 清肝经5分钟：

用拇指指腹从食指掌面指根直推至指尖。

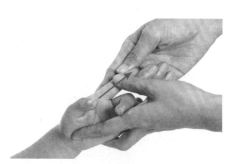

3. 清肺经5分钟：

用拇指指腹从无名指掌面指根直推至指尖。

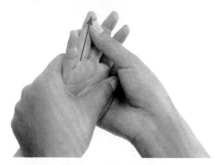

4. 揉阳池5分钟：

用拇指和中指指端相对用力揉手背一窝风上3寸凹陷处。

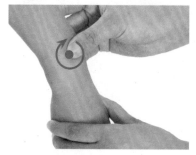

贴心提示

有鼻炎病史的孩子通常一感冒就犯鼻炎。要想控制鼻炎，预防感冒是关键，平时可经常搓一搓鼻翼两侧。

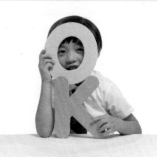

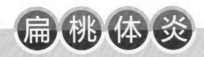

扁桃体炎

扁桃体炎多由于风热邪毒从口鼻而入，侵犯肺胃二经。咽喉为肺胃之门户，首当其冲，邪毒相搏，郁结于咽喉两旁所致。此病多为急性，多属实证。

手部穴位精解

清天河水

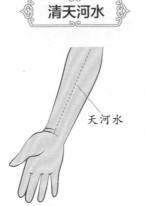

天河水

【准确定位】前臂内侧正中，总筋至洪池成一直线。

【按摩手法】一手握住小儿手，使掌心向上，用另一手食指和中指指腹自小儿腕横纹推向肘横纹。

【功效作用】清心除烦，镇惊安神，退热发表。

清胃经

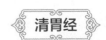
胃经

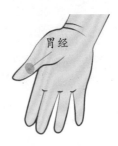

【准确定位】拇指掌面近掌端第一节。

【按摩手法】一手托住小儿手，使掌心向上，用另一手拇指指腹从小儿拇指掌根推至拇指指根。

【功效作用】清胃热，降胃气。

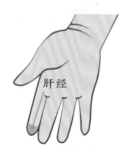

清肝经

肝经

【准确定位】食指掌面。

【按摩手法】一手托住小儿手，使掌心向上，用另一手拇指指腹从小儿食指指根直推至指尖。

【功效作用】清热，排毒。

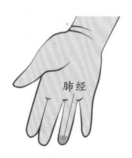

清肺经

肺经

【准确定位】无名指掌面。

【按摩手法】一手托住小儿手，使掌心向上，用另一手拇指指腹从小儿无名指指根直推至指尖。

【功效作用】宣肺清热，疏风解表，化痰止咳。

急性扁桃体炎

【症状表现】发热或高或低，咽痛，吞咽不利，有时伴烦躁、口干、便秘。

【治疗原则】清热解毒，利咽通腑。

【按摩频率】每天2次，5天为1个疗程。

1. 清天河水5分钟：

用食指和中指指腹自腕掌侧横纹推至肘横纹。

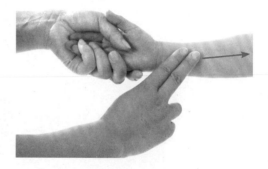

2. 清肝经5分钟：

用拇指指腹从食指掌面指根直推至指尖。

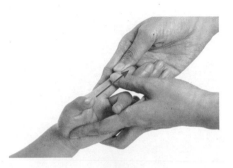

3. 清肺经5分钟：

用拇指指腹从无名指掌面指根直推至指尖。

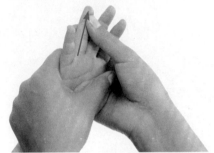

4. 清胃经5分钟：

用拇指指腹自拇指掌根推至拇指指根。

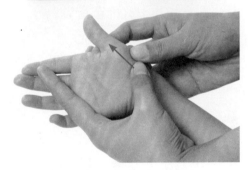

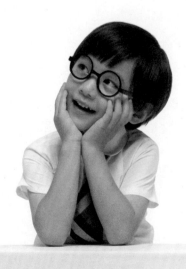

哮喘是一种发作性痰鸣气喘的疾病，以阵发性哮鸣气促、呼气延长为特征，多与肺、脾、肾三脏有关，其病机多为本虚标实，一般急性发作期以邪实为主，缓解期以正虚为主。

手部穴位精解

逆运八卦

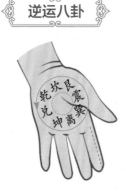

【准确定位】掌中，围绕掌心内劳宫一周，按乾、坎、艮、震、巽、离、坤、兑八卦分布。

【按摩手法】一手托住小儿手，使掌心向上，用另一手拇指指腹自小儿艮宫起逆时针做运法。

【功效作用】降气平喘。

揉外劳宫

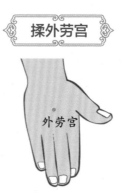

【准确定位】掌背正中，与内劳宫相对处。

【按摩手法】一手握住小儿手，使掌背向上，用另一手中指指端揉小儿本穴。

【功效作用】温阳散寒，升阳举陷，发汗解表。

推四横纹

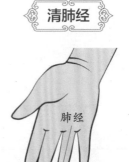

四横纹

【准确定位】掌面食指、中指、无名指、小指第一指间关节横纹处。

【按摩手法】一手持小儿手，使掌心向上，用另一手拇指指腹从小儿食指横纹推向小指横纹处，来回推。

【功效作用】调中行气，和气血，消胀满。

清肺经

肺经

【准确定位】无名指掌面。

【按摩手法】一手托住小儿手，使掌心向上，用另一手拇指指腹从小儿无名指指根直推至指尖。

【功效作用】宣肺清热，疏风解表，化痰止咳。

清天河水

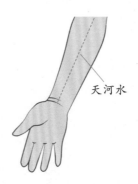

天河水

【准确定位】前臂内侧正中，总筋至洪池成一直线。

【按摩手法】一手握住小儿手，使掌心向上，用另一手食指和中指指腹自小儿腕横纹推向肘横纹。

【功效作用】清心除烦，镇惊安神，退热发表。

寒性哮喘

【症状表现】寒性，咳喘哮鸣，吐痰清稀，面色白，形寒怕冷。

【治疗原则】温肺化痰，降逆平喘。

【按摩频率】每天2次，5天为1个疗程。

1. 逆运八卦5分钟：

以拇指指腹自艮宫起逆时针做运法。

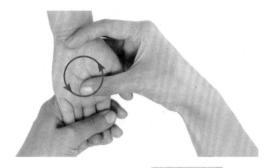

2. 揉外劳宫5分钟：

用中指指端揉掌背正中与内劳宫相对处。

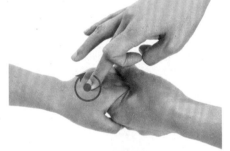

3. 推四横纹5分钟：

用拇指指腹从食指横纹推向小指横纹处，来回推。

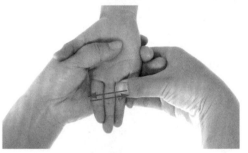

4. 清肺经5分钟：

用拇指指腹从无名指掌面指根直推至指尖。

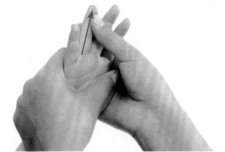

热性哮喘

【症状表现】热性，咳喘哮鸣，痰色黄稠，口干咽燥或有发热。缓解期，面色白，神疲乏力，自汗，食少便溏，形寒怕冷。

【治疗原则】清热化痰，降逆平喘；缓解期，健脾补肾纳气。

【按摩频率】每天2次，5天为1个疗程。

1. 逆运八卦5分钟：

以拇指指腹自艮宫起逆时针做运法。

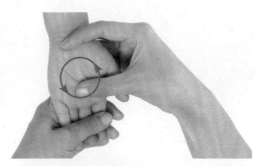

2. 清天河水5分钟：

用食指和中指指腹自腕掌侧横纹推至肘横纹。

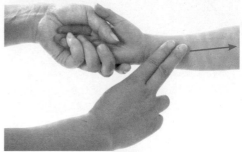

3. 推四横纹5分钟：

用拇指指腹从食指横纹推向小指横纹处，来回推。

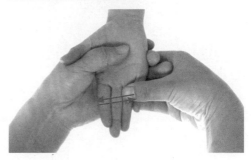

ORDER FORM

	Quantity	Cdn Price	U.S. Price	Total
Share The Fire	_____	$15.00	$12.00	_____
Pray With Fire	_____	$15.00	$12.00	_____
Catch the Fire	_____	$15.00	$12.00	_____
			Subtotal:	_____

Applicable Postage, Handling and Taxes will be added.

Fax your order to 905 847 7931.
Include your VISA number:

VISA # _____ exp _____

Signature _____

Name _____

Address _____

_____

**For quantity and bookstore discounts,
fax 905 847 7931**